Youcef Oussed...

Promoting a culture of patient safety

Youcef Oussama Fourar

Promoting a culture of patient safety

Models and Practices

ScienciaScripts

Imprint

Cover image: www.ingimage.com

This book is a translation from the original published under ISBN 978-620-6-69407-6.

Publisher:
Sciencia Scripts
is a trademark of
Dodo Books Indian Ocean Ltd. and OmniScriptum S.R.L publishing group

120 High Road, East Finchley, London, N2 9ED, United Kingdom
Str. Armeneasca 28/1, office 1, Chisinau MD-2012, Republic of Moldova, Europe

ISBN: 978-620-6-58783-5

Promoting a culture of patient safety

Models and Practices

TABLE OF CONTENTS

Introduction

The notion of SC first appeared in a report prepared by the International Nuclear Safety Advisory Group (INSAG) after the Chernobyl disaster. A low level of 'Safety Culture' was identified as one of the contributing factors to the worst nuclear accident in history. The years following the accident have seen a more widespread use of the concept of SC, particularly in high-risk industries, to explain a number of accidents (e.g. Bhopal, 1984; Chernobyl, 1986; Pier Alpha, 1988; Deepwater Horizon, 2010, etc.) due to organisational failures.

Thus, the concept of SC has been introduced to study the shared values, attitudes and behaviours that together proactively determine the predisposition of companies towards the deployment of safety promotion approaches, particularly in the healthcare field, where several attempts to apply this type of approach have failed. A high level of patient safety culture (PSC) is linked to a strong involvement of healthcare professionals in promoting safe care. This safety is often characterised by a reduction in the number of adverse events and, consequently, fewer medical errors and, consequently, an improvement in the quality and safety of care.

It is against this backdrop that this book explores the theoretical underpinnings of patient safety culture, presents practical methodologies for its enhancement and proposes concrete applications for improving the quality and safety of care. Drawing on extensive research, the book begins by elucidating the fundamental theories underpinning patient safety culture. It examines the relationship between organisational culture, human behaviour and patient safety, providing a sound theoretical framework to inform subsequent discussions.

Chapters 1 and 2 of the book provide a rich toolkit of strategies, methods and best practices to assess and measure patient safety culture, foster open communication, promote continuous learning and integrate safety practices into day-to-day healthcare operations. Chapters 3 and 4 present application-oriented approaches that ensure readers can translate theory and methodology into tangible improvements within healthcare organisations. They present case studies from Algerian healthcare settings, demonstrating how a strong patient safety culture can lead to a reduction in medical errors, increased staff engagement and improved quality and safety of care.

Ultimately, this book is a vital resource for healthcare professionals, administrators, policy makers and researchers dedicated to raising the standards of patient safety. It highlights the importance of nurturing a culture of safety as an integral part of healthcare delivery, with the overriding aim of protecting healthcare workers and patients and promoting excellence in healthcare systems. This book not only provides readers with the knowledge and tools to drive change, but also inspires a renewed commitment to making patient safety a top priority in healthcare organisations worldwide.

Chapter I

General information on safety culture

1.1. Introduction

The concept of safety culture (SC) was first introduced in an accident report prepared by the International Nuclear Safety Advisory Group (INSAG) after the Chernobyl disaster in 1986. A low level of 'safety culture' was identified as one of the contributing factors to the worst nuclear accident in history. As a result, SC and its manifestation in the form of safety climate have been the subject of much scientific research over the past 30 years, where a positive culture has been linked to better safety performance.

1.2. Concept of Culture

The concept of culture has begun to attract the attention of safety researchers since Turner's publication "*Man Made Disaster*" in which culture is discussed as a contributing factor to accidents (Goncalves Filho and Waterson 2018). Thus, in recent years, the focus on technical aspects and safety management systems as a means of ensuring safety has shifted to include cultural aspects (Besnard et al. 2018).

The study of culture has become essential because of its strong impact on human behaviour. It also explains the beliefs and values shared by the members of an organisation. This culture is built around the experiences of members of the same organisation. These experiences build knowledge that is then transformed into shared values and practices, which in turn help to create a culture that is often referred to as the organisational culture. (Guldenmund 2010).

1.3. Culture & Organisational Climate

The introduction of the concept of organisational culture has made it possible to integrate a new approach into the management of organisations. Managers now see human and organisational factors as determinants of the success or failure of their organisations. Controlling these factors can therefore help to improve the organisation's functions, particularly in the field of occupational health and safety (OHS). (Hudson 2007).

Similarly, the focus on human and organisational factors in OHS has led to the study of cultural factors that might influence the safety performance of organisations. This focus was underlined after the occurrence of a number of accidents affecting a wide range of industries (e.g. Bhopal, 1984; Chernobyl, 1986; Pier Alpha, 1988; Deepwater Horizon, 2010, etc.). (Kirwan, Reader, and Parand 2019).

The concept of safety culture was introduced to study the shared values, attitudes and behaviours that together proactively determine an organisation's safety performance. (Le Coze 2019). However, it is useful to first discuss the concept of organisational culture before venturing into the details of the concept of safety culture.

Indeed, the emergence of the concepts of organisational culture and organisational climate extended from the 1970s to the 1980s, when they developed successively rather than in parallel. A great deal of research was carried out in the 1970s under the term organisational climate, which then began to be gradually replaced in the 1980s by the term organisational culture (Guldenmund 2010).

Researchers have described them as 'umbrella' concepts because they give an abstract vision of the organisation, while no distinction can be made between them. (Schein 1992) is considered to be the first researcher to make a clear distinction between the two concepts by giving them appropriate definitions.

In this context, he explained that climate is a manifestation and reflection of cultural assumptions, meaning that organisational culture manifests itself through organisational climate. He reinforced this by giving an explicit definition of organisational culture:

"A pattern of shared basic assumptions that the group has learned in solving its problems of external adaptation and internal integration and that has worked well enough to be considered valid and, therefore, to be taught to new members as the right way to perceive, think and act in relation to these problems".   (Schein 1992)

This distinction between the concepts can also be made by the fact that organisational climate is often characterised by a limited dimensionality which can be measured by quantitative approaches using self-administered questionnaires. Whereas organisational culture is often determined phenomenologically by qualitative studies (e.g. observations, interviews, documentary analyses, etc.) (Antonsen 2017).

More elsewhere, (Guldenmund 2000) discussed the differences between organisational climate and organisational culture in more detail, where it was found that the term organisational climate was initially used to refer to a broader concept of underlying organisational events and processes. However, over time it has become linked solely to psychological or behavioural phenomena in an organisation.

Thus, the term culture was used to cover the global meaning that was previously covered by climate. This concept of organisational culture was defined as :

"A relatively stable, multidimensional, holistic construct shared by members (groups) of the organisation, which provides a frame of reference and gives meaning to / or is typically revealed in certain practices". (Guldenmund 2010)

In other words, culture is to a group what personality or character is to an individual. Just as our personality and character guide and constrain our behaviour, culture guides and constrains the observable behaviours of members of a group through the norms shared between them, which means that cultural characteristics explain different organisational behaviours and variance between levels of organisations (Schein and Schein 2017).

It should be noted that organisational culture is seen as the result of the ongoing interactions of three sources: (1) the views and values of the founder of the organisation; (2) the learning experiences of group members as their organisation gradually evolves; and (3) new values, beliefs and assumptions with which new members and leaders enter the organisation.

The interaction between these three elements is what contributes to the process of forming the values, attitudes and behaviours shared by the members of the organisation (Schein and Schein 2017). In addition, the manifestation of organisational culture can be explained through 3 layers which are from the deepest to the most superficial (Guldenmund 2000):

1. *The basic assumptions* that are unconscious, invisible and deeply rooted in the organisation, and which subsequently determine values and behaviour;
2. *Adopted values, which are* conscious and visible attitudes, values, norms and rules of behaviour that members use as a means of representing the culture to themselves and to others;
3. *Artefacts* form the visible part of the culture, translating earlier layers into direct manifestations.

So, this relationship between culture, behaviours and practices is what drives managers and researchers to place such importance on organisational culture and subsequently safety culture (Occelli 2018). This leads us to establish the link between organisational culture and safety culture.

1.4. Organisational culture and safety culture: what link?

Organisational culture has long been used by researchers and managers for its direct link to organisational performance. It has been established that a positive organisational culture leads to stronger organisational commitment, improved performance and generally higher productivity (Cooper 2000).

In addition, a company's organisational culture reflects the shared behaviours, beliefs, attitudes and values towards the objectives, functions and procedures related to all aspects of the organisation, including safety. However, the concept of organisational culture is holistic in the sense that it encompasses several facets of the organisation. It was therefore deemed necessary to introduce the concept of safety culture.

The concept of safety culture has therefore appeared in the scientific literature to analyse the safety aspect of an organisation. In other words, safety culture (SC) is a subset of organisational culture that makes it possible to study the shared values, attitudes and behaviours that together determine an organisation's safety performance.

1.5. Safety Culture

The concept of 'Safety Culture' (SC) was first used in 1984 after the Bhopal chemical plant explosion in India to show that the Indian national culture at that time was not conducive to safety. However, it was officially introduced in an accident report prepared by the International Nuclear Safety Group (INSAG) for the International Atomic Energy Agency (IAEA) after the Chernobyl disaster in 1986. A low level of 'safety culture' was identified as one of the contributing factors to the worst nuclear accident in history (INSAG 1986).

Since then, the concept of CS has begun to attract the attention of the scientific community where it has been argued that poor CS is one of the main causes of key accidents that have affected a wide range of industrial sectors (i.e. aviation, nuclear, petrochemical, rail, maritime, etc.). (Cox and Flin 1998; Kirwan et al. 2019; Silbey 2009). However, despite the wide use of the concept and the considerable literature covering its theoretical and empirical aspects, its definition remains one of the most debated topics in the scientific community (Cooper 2000).

In this regard, the Australian Centre for Research on Employment and Work published a systematic review of CS definitions in 2014 in which a number of 51 original definitions were found in the scientific literature from 1991 to 2013. However, only 24 of these were based on theoretical models (Vu and Cieri 2014).

This plethora of definitions can be explained by the fact that, at the beginning, CS did not have a solid theoretical foundation and was introduced to justify the occurrence of a number of accidents that affected various industries (Reiman and Rollenhagen 2014). Consequently, this situation of ambiguity has given researchers from all disciplines (e.g. psychology, sociology, anthropology, etc.) and industry professionals the opportunity to make numerous proposals to make the concept of CS more tangible (Cooper 2016).

In his literature review, (Guldenmund 2000) identified 7 definitions of SA which, according to him, are very implicit, with the exception of one which covers the key elements of SA very explicitly. This definition is the one provided by the UK Health and Safety Commission (HSC) for the Advisory Committee on Safety of Nuclear Installations (ACSNI):

"Safety culture is the product of individual and collective values, attitudes, perceptions, skills and patterns of behaviour that determine the commitment, style and effectiveness of an organisation's health and safety management". (ACSNI 1993)

For (Cooper, 2000)this definition is the most holistic because it highlights both the functionalist aspect of SC, where its predetermined objective is clearly

11

stated, and the interpretive aspect, where SC is considered to be the product of a dynamic and reciprocal relationship between three essential components: psychological, behavioural and situational.

More recently, (Daniellou, Simard and Boissières, 2010) have provided a definition of CS that is consistent with that provided by ACSNI and Cooper's interpretations:

"Safety culture is the set of practices developed and repeated by the main players involved, to control the risks of their job". (Daniellou, Simard and Boissières, 2010)

The term "*Practices*" used in the definition includes both ways of thinking about safety and ways of acting towards it. This can be explained by the fact that the way of thinking refers to the values, attitudes, beliefs and convictions that a group of people have with regard to safety, and which consequently translate into a certain number of safety behaviours in various work situations (i.e. ways of acting with regard to safety).

These behaviours may be influenced not only by the values shared within an organisation, but also by situational constraints which may lead an employee to work against his or her safety convictions in certain exceptional situations (e.g. deliberate non-compliance with safety rules in order to maintain production in the event of a staff shortage) (Daniellou et al. 2010).

Analysis of these definitions clearly shows that SC is the product of values, attitudes, perceptions and skills that translate into safety behaviours, which will eventually determine the effectiveness of OHS management within an organisation.

However, a controversy regarding the identification of the determinants of SC and how they interact, has persisted in the scientific community and resulted in the development of several conceptual frameworks and theoretical models of SC and the introduction of the concept of safety climate (Gilbert et al. 2018).

1.6. Safety climate

The introduction of the concept of safety climate has created controversy, where we can see that the two concepts (i.e. climate and culture) are invoked interchangeably in the literature (Griffin and Curcuruto 2016). To remedy this, (Cooper, 2016) proposed a framework to distinguish these concepts by stating that safety culture refers to an enduring atmosphere that impacts organisational safety management (i.e. how we do things around here), whereas safety climate reflects the shared perceptions of safety by employees within the organisation (i.e. what we think about safety now).

In this regard, (Zohar and Polachek, 2014) have defined safety climate as the set of perceptions shared by employees regarding safety. These perceptions are formed in the work environment, around safety-related policies, procedures and practices and their relationship to organisational characteristics (Flin et al. 2000; Zohar 2010).

To explain the relationship between safety climate, behaviour and safety performance, various models have been proposed (Vierendeels et al. 2018). (Griffin and Neal, 2000) confirmed, in their model of safety climate and performance, that organisational characteristics are antecedents of safety climate and that they directly affect individual behaviour and, consequently, safety performance (Silva, Lima, and Baptista 2004; Vierendeels et al. 2018).

The (Christian et al. 2009) of safety at work is consistent with this and confirms the influence of the safety climate on individual aspects and how these influence safety performance and outcomes. The authors specify that safety performance is linked to safety behaviour and that safety results are directly linked to frequency and severity rates.

In another study, (Fugas, Silva and Meliá, 2012) proposed a model that identified the influence of safety climate on compliance with safety procedures and proactive safety outcomes. It was found that proactive safety outcomes are the result of a combination of individual and situational factors, with the latter being directly influenced by the safety climate (Zohar 2010).

What is remarkable about all these models is that none of them has been able to identify the direct relationship between safety culture and safety climate. Other authors have proposed replacing the concepts of safety climate and safety culture with that of organisational culture without taking into account that this change would not only lead to another definitional controversy, but would also reduce the priority given to OHS at the organisational level (Cooper 2016; Giorgi, Lockwood, and Glynn 2015).

From the above, there is a tendency to believe that the concepts of safety culture and safety climate are similar, but the concept of safety culture is considered to be more comprehensive than that of safety climate, which is considered to be more superficial in that it aims to study employees' current beliefs about safety. We will therefore use the concept of safety culture for the remainder of this book.

1.7. Safety Culture Analysis

The concept of safety culture has not only created controversy over its definition, but also conflict over how to approach it, where two different currents exist in the literature: the interpretive current and the functionalist current.

1. *The interpretative current,* favoured by social scientists, treats the organisation as a culture, while cultural reality is socially constructed by those who are part of it (i.e. an organisation is culture). This current seeks to approach culture as a framework that conceptualises the organisation while inspecting the various phenomena. These phenomena stem from beliefs attributed by the members of an organisation to its constituent elements (e.g. structure, systems and tools). Thus, the ultimate objective is to understand the

dominant culture, not to evaluate it, using qualitative research methods and accepting that culture is unique in each organisation and therefore no comparative study is possible (Reiman and Rollenhagen 2014).

2. *The functionalist trend,* favoured by managers and practitioners, sees culture as a variable that can be designed and modified to achieve a set of objectives (i.e. an organisation has a culture). This culture manifests itself through artefacts that reflect not only the values adopted but also the underlying assumptions. Thus, an organisation is seen as having a developed culture once its core values and assumptions are widely shared by its members. Proponents of this approach use quantitative research methods, in particular questionnaires, to assess employees' perceptions of safety and to propose action plans to improve the existing culture, safety behaviour and, consequently, the OHS performance of an organisation.

According to Cooper (Cooper 2016)the interpretive and functionalist streams are just two sides of the same coin as they seek to understand CS while proposing solutions for improvement. The author mentioned that a pragmatic movement has emerged recently, which considers culture as a process rather than an entity and tries to understand what is happening in the organisation (Gilbert et al. 2018).

1.8. Safety Culture Models

In order to better understand the complex concept of CS, four influential models that define the main elements of CS while representing the relationships between them will be discussed. These are :

a. Reason's model of interdependent subcultures (1998) ;
b. Guldenmund's three-layer model (2000) ;
c. Cooper's reciprocity model (2000) ;
d. TEAM model by Vierendeels et al (2018).

a. Reason's model of interdependent subcultures (1998)

Based on an organisational analysis of accidents, (Reason 1998) proposed a model of SC based on 5 interdependent subcultures (**Figure 1.1**), in which SC is seen as the product of various other subcultures.

- *Informed Culture,* where operational risks are understood by all members of an organisation;
- *Reporting Culture*, based on the existence of a centralised data collection system for reporting accidents and near misses;
- *Learning Culture*, which aims to analyse the data reported while learning lessons and disseminating knowledge within the organisation;
- *Flexible Culture*, which will evolve according to the knowledge acquired during the learning process;
- *Just* Culture, which is considered to be at the heart of the whole learning process, i.e. without '*Just Culture*' there will be no accident reporting and no learning, and therefore no informed organisation.

The functionalist approach of Reason's model helps to guide organisations in their quest to prevent accidents at work by focusing on 5 different sub-cultures which are interdependent and which serve the same objective of developing a CS.

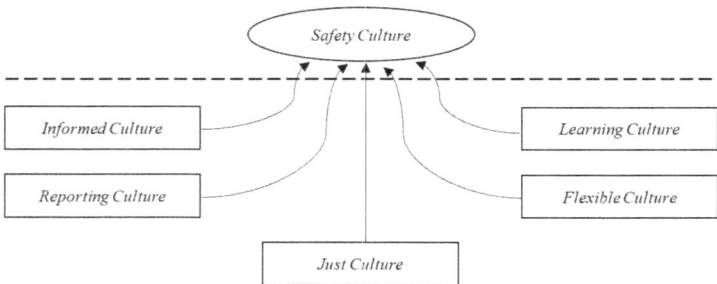

Figure 1.1: Reason's 1998 model of interdependent subcultures.

b. Guldenmund's three-layer model (2000)

Based on Schein's interpretive model of organisational culture (Schein 1992), (Guldenmund 2000) proposed a three-layer model of SC (**Figure 1.2**). These layers are from the deepest to the most superficial:

- *The basic assumptions* that are unconscious, invisible, and are considered to be the triggers of safety behaviours;
- *The values adopted, which are* visible conscious attitudes that directly affect four major categories of security objects (i.e. hardware, software, people, behaviour);
- *Artefacts*, which form the visible part of the culture, translate the previous deep layers into direct manifestations (e.g. wearing PPE).

This model suffers from major shortcomings, as it approaches SA in an interpretive way where the focus is on understanding the dominant culture in an organisation and its effect on staff attitudes using safety surveys. Thus, SC is only understood through the assessor's analysis of the data collected and, in some cases, through interviews, observations and focus groups, which is considered an incomplete understanding of the culture.

Furthermore, there is no clear taxonomy of core assumptions and their identification relies solely on the agreement of organisational members (Cooper 2016). This model also assumes a simple cause-effect relationship and a unidirectional relationship between core assumptions and artefacts, which are considered ineffective in accident prevention (Lund and Aarø 2004).

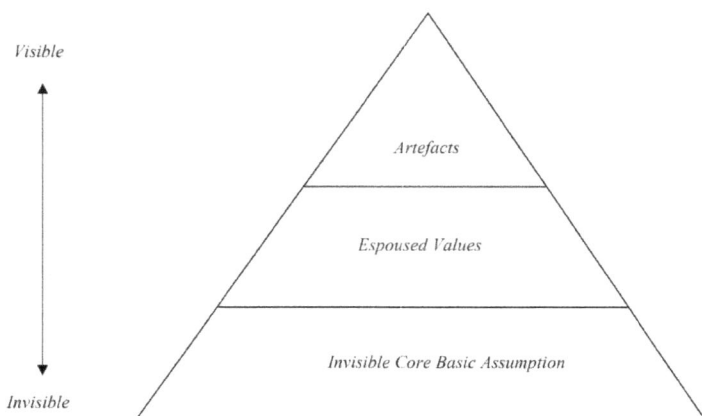

Figure 1.2: Guldenmund 2000 three-layer model.

c. Cooper's reciprocity model (2000)

Based on the reciprocal determinism model of (Bandura 1986) proposed in the social cognitive theory(Cooper, 2000) proposed a reciprocal model of SA (**Figure 1.3**), which contains three factors:

- *Internal psychological factors*, which refer to subjective attitudes and perceptions and can be measured using safety climate questionnaires;
- *External safety behaviours* that can be observed and improved through behavioural safety initiatives;
- *Objective situational characteristics* that involve not only a procedural aspect (e.g. operating procedures, communication flow and safety management systems) that can be assessed using safety audits and inspections, but also technical aspects such as the design of the production system and environmental aspects (e.g. noise, heat, lighting) (Vierendeels et al. 2018).

The functionalist approach of Cooper's model provides a better understanding of safety culture, because it is seen as the product of dynamic reciprocal relationships between three constituent aspects (i.e. psychological, behavioural and situational).

This dynamic relationship provided a holistic view of the construction of the SC and, as a result, enabled improvement actions to be better targeted. This model was then transformed into a business process model of (Cooper, 2002) where the psychological, behavioural and situational aspects were considered as inputs that would be transformed into objectives and management practices for the organisation.

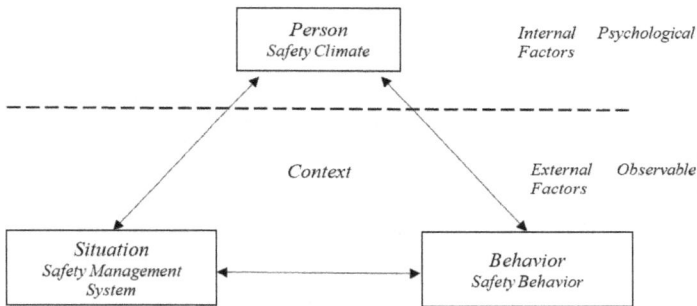

Figure 1.3. Cooper 2000 reciprocity model.

d. TEAM model by Vierendeels et al (2018)

Based on a thorough review of influential models of safety culture and safety climate that have been proposed in the literature, (Vierendeels et al. 2018) constructed a three-layer integrative model of SC called the 'Egg Aggregated Model-TEAM' (**Figure 1.4**). This model provides a holistic view of all aspects that can influence the safety of an organisation while taking into account their interrelationships. The model is composed of three layers or domains:

- *Technological area of* observable factors that can be measured using safety indicators (e.g. frequency rate, severity rate, safety audits, etc.);

- *Organisational aspect of* the safety climate: perceptual and personal psychological factors measured using safety climate questionnaires;
- Personal *psychological domain of* motivation and behaviour that can also be measured using questionnaires.

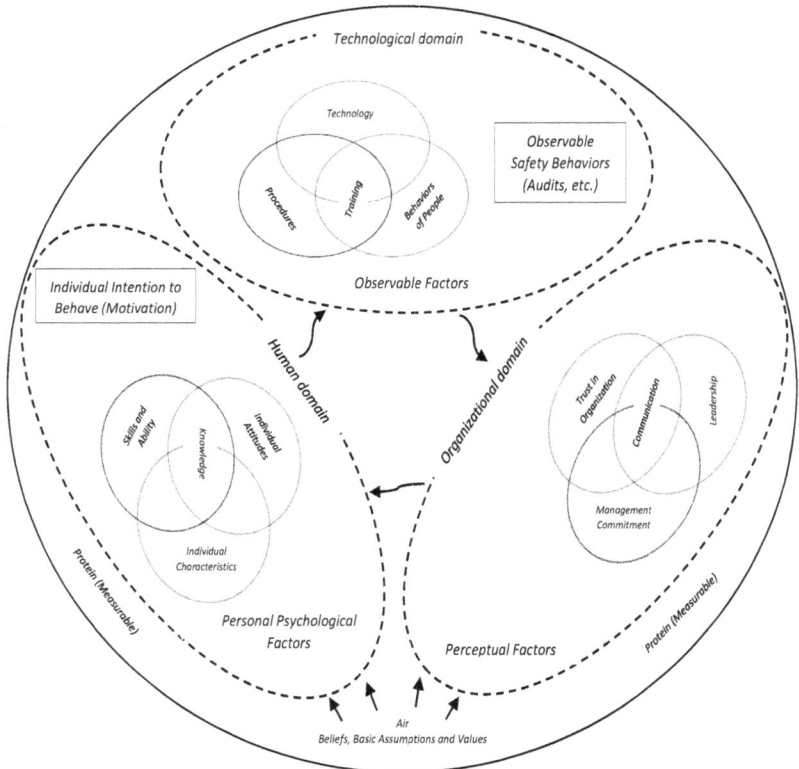

Figure 1.4. TEAM model from Vierendeels et al 2018.

The authors referred to the shape of the egg and its components as a form of metaphor to distinguish between observable and non-observable parts, in order to better explain the visibility of each layer of the SC and the relationships between them. Fundamental values, beliefs and assumptions can be represented by the air in the egg, which is invisible but an essential part of it. This model is considered to be the most holistic as it integrates both culture and safety climate while representing the reciprocal relationships that exist between them.

An analysis of the various models shows that the emphasis is on the observable part of safety culture, often referred to as the safety climate. The various components of these models are often used by researchers to define the dimensions of safety culture that will be capitalised on to develop what are known as safety climate questionnaires. This approach to studying safety culture using questionnaires is called the dimensional approach.

1.9. Conclusion

Throughout this chapter, a review has been made of safety culture: its origins, its links with organisational culture and the safety climate. This analysis shows that SC was first used in the industrial sector to investigate a number of accidents that occurred because of organisational deficiencies. It is seen as a proactive indicator of safety performance. As a result, the evaluation of CS has become a priority for organisations where there are two currents in the scientific literature, the interpretative current and the functionalist current.

What is important to highlight about this functionalist trend and its approaches is that it was adopted in the healthcare sector after the appearance of the Institute of Medicine report, which highlighted the importance of promoting a culture of safety in the healthcare sector. As a result, Patient Safety Culture (PSC) assessment has become a management tool used by managers in healthcare organisations. It has multiple benefits: raising staff awareness, assessing the current state of patient safety, evaluating the impact of interventions to improve patient safety and benchmarking.

Chapter II

Patient Safety Culture

2.1. Introduction

The importance attached to safety in the healthcare sector has always been linked to the prevention of adverse events, which are considered a global concern and where statistics show that significant percentages of patients receiving treatment have experienced some sort of adverse event during their admission cycle (e.g. USA 4%, UK 10%, Canada 7.5% and Australia 16.6%) (Pronovost et al. 2011).

This situation was further exacerbated by the appearance of the groundbreaking report "*To Err is Human*" by the Institute of Medicine (IOM) in 1999, which triggered a global awareness of healthcare safety. Several international projects were launched, including the World Health Organization-World Alliance on Patient Safety Project and the Organization for Economic Cooperation and Development (OECD - Healthcare Quality Indicator Project) (Kohn, Corrigan, and Molla 1999; Wischet and Schusterschitz 2009).

As a result, the healthcare sector began to look for systemic remedial solutions to adverse events. These solutions have been found in the theories of safety science, given the similarities that exist between industrial organisations and healthcare establishments.

This quest has also led to the consideration of cultural aspects as latent factors in adverse events and causes of accidents and has prompted researchers not only to adopt the concept of safety culture in the healthcare sector under the concept of "Care Safety Culture", but also to adopt appropriate methods to study, evaluate and subsequently improve them (Benzer, Meterko, and Singer 2017).

The importance of cultural aspects has also been reinforced by a number of studies that have shown a positive correlation between safety culture, implementation of safety practices and improved patient safety (Xuanyue et al. 2013).

In this regard, (Braithwaite et al. 2017) conducted a systematic literature review to investigate the link between organisational culture and patient safety performance. The study included 62 articles of which 94% were quantitative, 81% were cross-sectional and only 4% were interventional. A positive association between organisational culture and patient safety performance was found in 48.4% of the studies and considering that PSC is embedded in the broader concept of organisational culture.

2.2. Patient Safety Culture

It is important to remember that care safety refers to the prevention and improvement of adverse outcomes or injuries resulting from care processes (Goh, Chan, and Kuziemsky 2013).

This improvement is linked to a healthcare organisation's safety culture, which is a crucial factor in the success of its safety and quality improvement initiatives (Speroff et al. 2010). Thus, having a culture that promotes safety within an organisation is an essential and substantial precursor to improving patient safety.

Consequently, the concept of PSC has been used in the healthcare sector to deal with that part of organisational culture which is concerned with safety aspects in healthcare organisations. Before attempting to define it, it is worth recalling the definition of safety culture as proposed by (Cooper, 2016) :

"The observable degree of effort e with which all members of the organisation direct their attention and actions towards improving day-to-day safety". (Cooper, 2016)

This definition highlights the proactive aspect with a specific aim and the way in which people think and behave with regard to safety. The construction of the PSC concept focuses directly on the organisation and individual activities aimed at improving safety, a variable that can be regularly monitored over time (i.e. evaluation of the effort that people devote to safety). This product is used in the field of PSC in a way that contributes to the development of SC (Vogus and Sutcliffe 2007).

However, there has been little consensus on the definition of patient safety culture (PSC) since it was first used. According to The European Society for Quality in Health Care, PSC is defined as follows:

"An integrated model of individual and organisational behaviour, based on shared beliefs and values, that continuously seeks to minimise the harm that patients may experience as a result of care delivery processes". (Wischet and Schusterschitz, 2009)

In other words, PSC is used as a means of managing risks and improving the quality of care, and this translates into consistency in policies, procedures and practices, as well as integration of the issue of care safety at all levels of an organisation.

2.3. Analysis of patient safety culture

There are 2 main approaches to detailed analysis of SSC, namely the typological and dimensional approaches.

2.3.1. Typological approach

Cultural maturity models enable organisations to be classified according to their levels of process maturity into predefined categories using a set of multidimensional criteria. (Pullen 2007) proposed the following definition:

"A maturity model is a structured set of elements that describe the characteristics of effective processes at different stages of development. It also suggests demarcation points between stages and methods of transition from one stage to another".   (Pullen 2007)

Maturity models have been used in a number of areas such as IT, information management and security management (Wendler 2012). In the latter case, cultural maturity models consist of classifying organisations using a continuum ranging from pathological organisations (i.e. non-existent culture) on the one hand to generative organisations (i.e. continuous improvement culture) on the other, passing through intermediate levels where organisations act in reaction to security or on a proactive basis (i.e. Calculative, Reactive and Proactive organisations) (Goncalves Filho and Waterson 2018).

Safety Culture Maturity Models (SCMMs) can be used as an assessment tool where a combination of methods is deployed to determine an organisation's level of maturity (e.g. focus groups, interviews, questionnaires, etc.).

This assessment can be constructed using a matrix in which each cell contains a description of the main performance characteristics, enabling different levels of maturity to be identified and organisations to be ranked accordingly. After that, MMCS becomes an improvement tool by identifying gaps and proposing action plans to improve the organisation's CS and consequently advance its position in the cultural ladder (Stemn et al. 2019).

The use of cultural maturity models as a CS assessment tool can be traced back to two main origins, namely the Quality Management Maturity Grid (QMMG) and Westrum's typology of organisational culture:

1. *Quality Management Maturity Grid (QMMG)*, proposed by Crosby in 1979, the QMMG has been used to establish the fact that an organisation must pass through five successive levels of quality maturity (i.e. Uncertainty, Awakening, Enlightenment, Wisdom and Certainty) in order to reach the total quality level of its activities (María R. Calingo 1996; Wendler 2012).

   The QMMG was then adapted to software engineering and became the Capability Maturity Model (CMM) composed of five maturity levels (i.e. Initial, Repeatable, Defined, Managed and Optimizing), which must first be identified in order to guide software improvement actions (Paulk et al. 1993).

2. *Westrum's typology of organisational culture*, consisting of three levels, has made it possible to classify organisations according to their culture into (1) Pathological culture, in which only individual power is considered; (2) Bureaucratic culture, in which only rules, positions and responsibilities are taken into account; (3) Generative culture, in which all the emphasis is placed on the mission itself and not on people or positions. (Westrum 1993, 2004).

Westrum's typology is based on the way in which organisations manage the flow of information, particularly that relating to anomalies (Parker, Lawrie, and Hudson 2006; Westrum 2004) :

- *In pathological organisations,* information is hidden to cover up failure or to be used as a personal resource in political power struggles.
- *Bureaucratic organisations:* information is collected and transmitted via standard channels, which slows down the process, particularly in crisis situations;
- *Generative organisations* are always looking for relevant information that will be communicated to the right person in the right form at the right time, while encouraging people to report anomalies as part of a continuous learning process;

According to (Goncalves Filho and Waterson, 2018)this typology has been adopted in several sectors (e.g. petrochemicals, health, food, aviation, construction, nuclear, etc.) and is considered to be the basis of the best-known maturity models such as themodel (Hudson 2007) used in the petrochemical industry and the Manchester Patient Safety Assessment Framework (MaPSaF) used in the healthcare sector (Ashcroft et al. 2005).

The most influential models in the literature include :

1. Bradley's cultural maturity model (1994);
2. Fleming's cultural maturity model (2000);
3. Hudson's cultural maturity model (2007);
4. Simard's Cultural Maturity Model (2018).

In order to better understand the theoretical underpinnings and to make the link with PSC, each model will be discussed in detail.

a. Bradley's cultural maturity model (1994)

In the 1990s, the chemical company 'DuPont' launched a project aimed at finding solutions to encourage continuous improvement in safety within their organisation. The project resulted in the proposal of a safety culture maturity model (**Figure 2.1**) called the 'Bradley Curve'.[Behari 2019; DuPontTM 2009].

The curve assumes that accident rates decrease with positive CS which, in turn, is directly related to the type of leadership, creating 4 progressive types of CS:

- *Reactive*, accidents are seen as an unavoidable part of day-to-day activities and no commitment to safety is shown by managers or employees;
- *Dependant*, safety is imposed by technical and procedural aspects, employees are obliged to follow safety rules, while accidents are considered to be caused by the violation of these rules ;

- Management assumes full responsibility for safety while encouraging employee participation in the process of finding solutions;
- *Interdependently*, safety is managed collectively by managers and employees, where communication, training and participation are seen as key aspects of successful safety management.

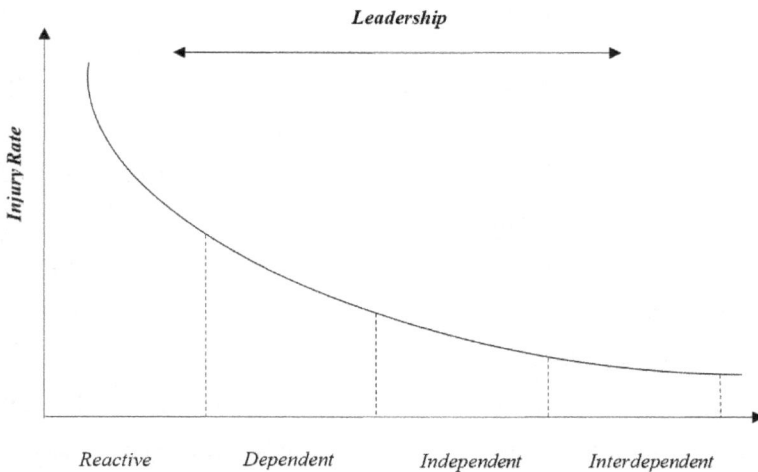

Figure 2.1. Cultural maturity model from Bradley 1994.

b. Fleming's cultural maturity model (2000)

In a report by the Health & Safety Executive (HSE), (Fleming 2000) proposed a 5-level safety culture maturity model. This model was developed on the basis of a review of previous models (e.g. Bradley model) and by holding discussions with the main safety managers in the industry.

It was found that safety culture maturity can be determined using 10 key elements (1) management commitment, (2) communication, (3) production versus safety, (4) learning organisation, (5) safety resources, (6) participation, (7) shared perceptions of safety, (8) trust, (9) industrial relations and job satisfaction and (10) training.

The average maturity of these ten key elements is calculated in order to position an organisation's SC according to the 5 levels of maturity (**Figure 2.2**), which are (Cooper 2016; Fleming 2000) :

- *Emerging*, safety is not a priority for the organisation and is only defined by technical, procedural and regulatory aspects;
- *Managing*, management efforts are geared towards accident prevention by focusing on reducing dangerous behaviour;
- *Involving*, root cause analyses of accidents are carried out, workers are involved in the safety management process and safety performance is monitored using reactive indicators;
- *At Cooperating,* safety is seen as an important aspect of the overall structure of the organisation, all staff are treated equally and safety performance and safety information are managed effectively;
- *Continuous improvement*, accident prevention is a core organisational value where safety performance is constantly monitored using reactive and proactive indicators, innovative risk mitigation solutions are constantly considered and the quality of life of staff is monitored and improved.

After assigning the level of maturity of the safety culture, (Fleming 2000) insists on using a step-by-step approach to improvement in order to advance the organisation's position on the cultural ladder. He emphasised that the model refers to the maturity of behaviours and not that of OHS management systems.

The model is therefore relevant for use in organisations where the procedural and technical aspects of safety are working well, while accidents are mainly due to behavioural and cultural factors. The model has been validated by (Lardner, Fleming and Joyner, 2002) in a study involving a large petrochemical organisation in the UK. The maturity levels found were 'Involving' and 'Cooperating', reinforcing the fact that CS varies from site to site within the same organisation (Foster and Hoult 2013).

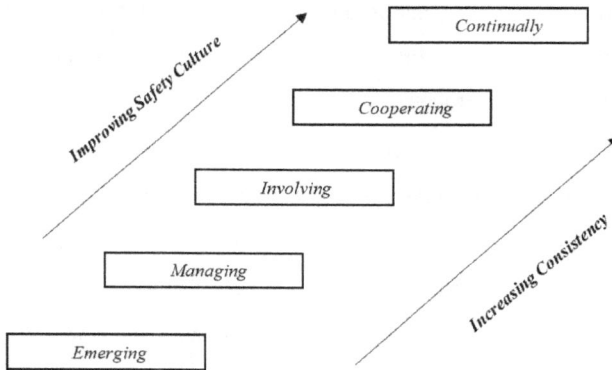

Figure 2.2. Fleming's cultural maturity model, 2000.

c. Hudson's cultural maturity model (2007)

Based on Westrum's typology, (Hudson 2007) proposed a 5-level cultural maturity model that allows organisations to move from the least to the most developed CS. The advantage of this model is that 2 levels of maturity have been added (i.e. *Proactive* and *Reactive*) and the *'Bureaucratic'* level has been replaced by the *'Calculative'* level. The aim of this move from 3 to 5 levels is to create a progressive scale that facilitates the process of improving CS (**Figure 2.3**).

The five-level typology of safety culture presented in this model consists of 5 categories of culture (Hudson 2007) :

- *Pathologically*, production is the number one priority and accidents are considered to be caused by employees;
- *Reactive*, safety is only taken into consideration after an accident has occurred;
- *Calculatively*, safety is enforced through safety management systems as a means of complying with regulations and avoiding penalties;
- *Proactive*, initiatives are being taken to involve operational staff in the safety process while reducing *top-down* approaches;
- *Generative*, safety is considered as an inherent aspect of organisations, while insisting on the involvement of all players at all levels of the organisation in this process.

To position organisations in the Hudson model, a framework of 18 elements ranging from concrete elements (safety management systems) to abstract elements (attitudes and behaviours) was developed, while providing a set of questions for each element to determine its level of maturity. The advantage of this model is that it can be applied to organisations with weaker safety management systems, unlike Fleming's model, which requires the existence of strong procedural and technical aspects of safety (Foster and Hoult 2013; Parker et al. 2006).

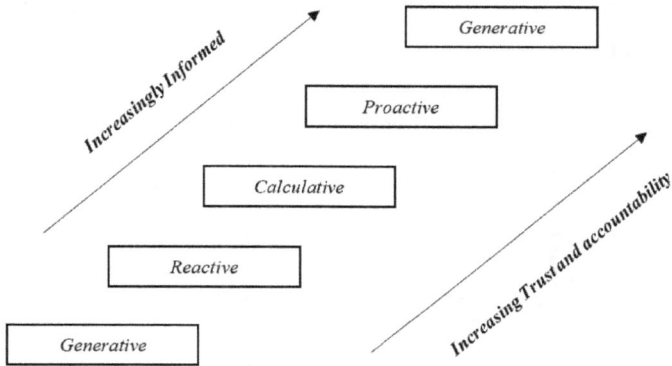

Figure 2.3. Hudson 2007 cultural maturity model.

d. Simard's Cultural Maturity Model (2010)

The (Daniellou, Simard and Boissières, 2010) assumes that SC is built around manager/employee interactions and the importance attached to safety in their decisions. Both groups are supposed to be involved in the safety process, but each of them may be more or less involved, thus creating a 4-level typology of SC **(Figure 2.4)**:

- As a *fatalist*, accidents are considered inevitable and cannot be prevented;
- Safety is considered to be the responsibility of employees who develop certain practices to protect themselves in situations not covered by safety rules;
- *In managerial terms*, safety is seen as the responsibility of management, which plays a major role in developing and implementing technical and procedural aspects in a formalised manner, while imposing them directly on employees without any prior involvement;

33

- *Integrated*, safety is managed using both a *'Top-down'* approach to apply safety guidelines and procedures, and a *'Bottom-up'* approach to progressively involve workers in the continuous improvement process (Besnard et al. 2018).

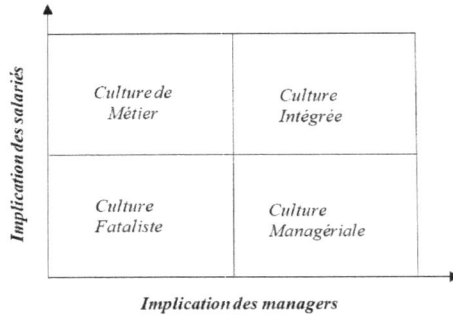

Implication des salariés

| Culture de Métier | Culture Intégrée |
| Culture Fataliste | Culture Managériale |

Implication des managers

Figure 2.4. Cultural maturity model from Simard 2018.

It should be noted that the 4 models presented above (**Figures 2.1 to 2.4**) have the same objective, which is to guide organisations in the process of improving their CS or CSP, which has always been linked to better safety performance (Stemn et al. 2019).

2.3.2. The Dimensional Approach

In the study of CS, safety culture/climate questionnaires are considered to be the predominant measurement instrument for assessing shared safety attitudes across the organisation. Questionnaires are often composed of a series of questions (i.e. items) that tap employees' perceptions of various aspects (i.e. dimensions, facets) considered relevant to safety. These dimensions may be either factors likely to cause accidents or key factors in their prevention (Noort et al. 2016).

The widespread use of questionnaires is due to the fact that self-administered questionnaires can be distributed to large groups of people in a relatively short space of time, providing instant quantitative results that allow the researcher to produce medians or averages, compare sub-groups and carry out benchmarking.

This assessment provides a proactive means of developing safety performance. This is because it identifies trends that are promising (e.g. shared beliefs about risk) and problematic (e.g. lack of incident reporting) for OHS management management (Halligan and Zecevic 2011; Noort et al. 2016)..

It should also be noted that there is a great deal of research on safety culture using different types of questionnaires, but we will confine ourselves to discussing just one questionnaire for illustrative purposes. This is the Nordic Safety Climate Questionnaire-50 (NOSACQ-50), which is regarded as a reliable instrument for measuring safety climate. It has been translated into several languages and has proved useful for predicting safety motivation, behaviour and performance. It consists of 50 items divided into 7 dimensions. Responses are assessed on a 4-point Likert-type scale 'strongly disagree, disagree, agree and strongly agree' (Kines et al. 2011; Yousefi et al. 2016).

Furthermore, the majority (94%) of studies on CS in the care sector have used quantitative methods, including self-administered questionnaires (Reis, Paiva, and Sousa 2018). Thus, it can be concluded that the study of SC in the healthcare sector falls within the *'functionalist stream'* discussed in the previous chapter.

On this subject, (Halligan and Zecevic, 2011) found in a literature review that included 139 studies of PSC that 126 of them used quantitative methods, mainly self-administered questionnaires, to assess PSC and the remaining 13 used qualitative analyses. (e.g. focus groups, observations and interviews) or a combination of qualitative and quantitative methods.

This observation prompted us to align ourselves with this trend by favouring an evaluation of PSC in the Algerian context by means of a quantitative assessment. More specifically, by using the dimensional approach to PSC. In this respect, the choice of using questionnaires as a tool for investigating PSC can be explained by its feasibility and its ability to collect a maximum amount of information in a minimum amount of time and with the least amount of effort, as well as ensuring the anonymity of respondents (Reis et al. 2018).

The dimensions measured are linked to factors that may contribute to the occurrence of accidents or to elements that play a role in their prevention. Each dimension is explored by a number of items that can be assessed by the responding sample using different types of scales (e.g. nominal, ordinal, etc.), then the responses are statistically processed to obtain an overall percentage of positive responses for each dimension that will show the most and least developed (Reis et al. 2018).

The literature review by(Halligan and Zecevic, 2011) showed that among the 12 questionnaires developed for the healthcare sector between 1980 and 2009, the number of dimensions varied between 3 and 12 and the number of items between 30 and 79; this means that no consensus was reached on the number of dimensions used or their names. Of these questionnaires, only four were the most frequently cited (**Table 2.1**): Hospital Survey on Patient Safety Culture - HSOPSC- (12 Dimensions), Safety Attitudes Questionnaire -SAQ- (6 Dimensions), Patient Safety Culture in Healthcare Organizations Survey -PSCHOS- (9 Dimensions) and Stanford Patient Safety Culture Survey Instrument -SPSCSI- (5 Dimensions).

Table 2.1. Dimensions measured by the 4 CSP questionnaires.

Questionnaire	Dimensions
HSOPSC	1. General perceptions of patient safety
	2. Frequency of events reported
	3. Supervisor/manager expectations and actions to promote patient safety
	4. Organisational learning - Continuous improvement
	5. Teamwork within the units
	6. Opening of communications
	7. Non-punitive response to an error
	8. Staffing
	9. Management support for patient safety
	10. Teamwork between units
SAQ	1. Teamwork climate
	2. Safety climate
	3. Job satisfaction
	4. Recognising stress
	5. Management perceptions
	6. Working conditions
PSCHO	1. Senior management commitment
	2. Organisational resources for safety
	3. General focus on safety
	4. Unit safety standards
	5. Recognition of unity and support for safety efforts
	6. Fear of shame
	7. Providing safe care
	8. Learning
	9. Fear of blame
MSI PSC	1. Organisational leadership in safety
	2. Unit leadership for safety
	3. Perceived state of safety
	4. Shame and repercussions of reporting
	5. Learning behaviour

Furthermore, it should be emphasised that the use of one of these questionnaires in a study can be explained by the validity of its psychometric properties, its relevance to the context studied and the sample measured. In this respect, it should be noted that the HSOPSC questionnaire was first developed in 2004 under the supervision of the American Agency of Healthcare Research (Sorra, Gray and Streagle, 2016; Badr, AlFadalah and El- Jardali, 2017) and has already been tested and validated in the United States, where it is widely used. It was then translated, tested and validated in 2013 by the Comité de Coordination de l'Evaluation Clinique et de la Qualité en Aquitaine-France (Occelli et al. 2013).

As a result, and in addition to its strong psychometric properties, the HSOPSC has become the most widely used instrument for assessing PSC (Tlili et al. 2020). For example, (Dunstan, Cook and Coyer, 2019) found in a review of PSC studies from 2010 to 2017 that the HSOPSC was the most widely used questionnaire in Australia.

In addition, HSOPSC is the best known questionnaire in the healthcare sector where it has been used in over 60 countries and translated into 36 languages (Reis et al. 2018). Its strong psychometric properties make it a reliable measurement tool in different contexts (Tlili et al. 2020).

As a reminder, this questionnaire is organised in two sections: the first section, relating to general information, is made up of five questions, while the second section explores staff perceptions of the UMC in their work unit. This second section is made up of 38 items organised into ten dimensions (**Table 2.1**).

Hospital professionals' responses to the questionnaire are recorded on a 5-point scale ranging from (5) strongly agree to (1) strongly disagree. Scores 4 and 5 are considered "positive" in relation to CS, score 3 is "neutral" and scores 1 and 2 are considered "negative." (Boughaba et al. 2019).

2.4. Discussion of the Dimensional Approach

The assessment of PSC using questionnaires was considered to be subjective, as it can be influenced by a number of uncontrolled factors. However, given the large number of respondents, this subjectivity is systematically cancelled out because it is calculated as an average over the large number of responses.

Some authors have criticised the fact that questionnaires have failed to expose the core of PSC, meaning that if we refer to Guldenmund's model of SC, questionnaires can at best investigate artefacts and espoused values but not core assumptions (Guldenmund 2010).

Bearing in mind that the questionnaires are designed to study perceptions considered to reflect workers' attitudes to safety. These attitudes are affected by the organisational context created by the policies drawn up at organisational level. Thus, workers can easily perceive and evaluate the impact of safety policies on their well-being and on the overall values attached to their safety. From this perspective, safety climate (attitudes) and PSC are not separate entities, but rather different approaches with the same objective, which is to determine the importance of safety within an organisation (Cooper 2016).

Based on this observation, we can state that the use of questionnaires is more than recommended to have a proactive vision of the current state of the PSC in order to better guide decision-making and the development of intervention plans to improve safety performance. To develop this type of questionnaire, two approaches are used: a theoretical approach in which a descriptive model of the safety climate is used, and a pragmatic approach in which the results of previous research can be combined to construct a new questionnaire. (Guldenmund 2010).

2.5. Conclusion

In this chapter, we will present the concept of PSC and the approaches to its analysis in order to understand the methodological discussions on measuring PSC using questionnaires or the Safety Culture Maturity Model (SCMM), which will be presented in chapters 3 and 4.

Chapter III

Contribution of Questionnaires to the Study of PSC

3.1. Introduction

In healthcare, the use of the concept of CS is part of the functionalist trend, which assumes the influence of culture on behaviour and subsequently on the results of care. Consequently, the existence of a positive CS translates into the presence of a set of observable behaviours that can improve the safety and quality of care.

As a result, assessing Patient Safety Culture (PSC) has become a priority for healthcare organisations. To do this, perceptions are assessed using self-administered questionnaires. This dimensional approach is the most widely used in the healthcare sector, followed by the typological approach, which ranks organisations on a scale of cultural maturity.

3.2. Contribution to the evaluation of the PSC in a Health Establishment

In order to justify the interest given to the quantitative evaluation (i.e. dimensional approach) of PSC in Algerian hospitals, we recall that the specialised literature shows that strategies for promoting the safety of care are based on two main objectives, which are the development of PSC and the continuous improvement of the quality and safety of care (Lee et al. 2015; Leggat and Balding 2018; Shaw-Taylor 2014).

Achieving the first objective, which is to promote safe care, depends on an evaluation of the PSC, with the aim of identifying the factors that hinder its promotion. This evaluation is based on three complementary aspects that define the complex concept of PSC (Cooper 2016) These are: the psychological aspect, which reflects how healthcare professionals feel; the behavioural aspect, which is inherent in practices in the field; and the situational aspect, which highlights an institution's policy on healthcare safety.

These three aspects are incorporated into the HSOPSC questionnaire, which is organised into two sections (**Appendix 1**): the first section, relating to general information, is made up of five questions, while the second section explores staff perceptions of PSC in their establishment.

It should also be remembered that for section 2, which is made up of ten dimensions, the dimensional score is obtained by dividing the total number of positive responses to questions in this dimension by the total number of responses to these questions:

$$S_{D_i} = \frac{np_i}{N_i} \; ; \; i = 1...10 \tag{3.1}$$

With : S_{D_i} being the score for the i dimension of the CS, np_i is the number of positive responses for this i dimension and N_i is the total number of responses for this i dimension, including positive, negative and neutral responses.

Consequently, a dimension is said to be developed if it has a score of 75% or more, whereas if the dimension has a score of 50% or less, it is said to be undeveloped. Finally, dimensions with scores between 50% and 75% are considered underdeveloped (Reis et al. 2018).

The HSOPSC questionnaire can be used to identify the problem areas in PSC and then draw up action plans to promote the safety and quality of care.

3.2.1. Materials & Methods

As indicated in the previous section, the aim of this study is to quantitatively evaluate the PSC of an Algerian hospital using the HSOPSC questionnaire. The recommended approach is that proposed by (Goodrick 2014) which we have adapted to the case of PSC measurement (**Figure 3.1**) (Boughaba et al. 2019).

1- Preparing the study on measuring PSC

↓

2- Distribution of questionnaires and data processing

↓

3- Capitalising on the results and proposing action plans

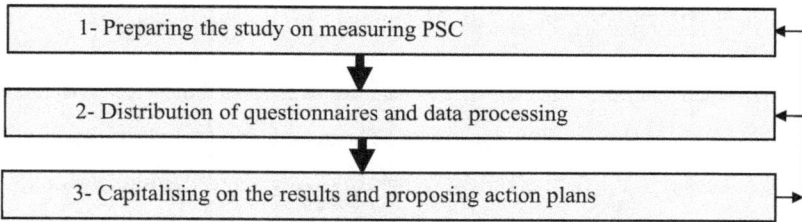

Figure 3.1: Stages in the recommended approach to assessing PSC.

In the first stage, a pilot hospital was chosen to carry out the first evaluation of PSC in the NHS. The questionnaire was distributed at the pilot hospital to 114 healthcare professionals who were selected by stratified random sampling in order to respect the distribution of the hospital's actual workforce, which is around 634 employees.

Stratified sampling is a method that involves first subdividing the population into homogeneous groups (strata) and then extracting a random sample from each stratum (occupational category). This method presupposes knowledge of the structure of the population. Various statistical formulas can be used to calculate the appropriate sample size with a controlled degree of confidence.

In this study, we used the following formulation of the sample size n :

$$
n = \frac{N\left(Z_{\left(1-\frac{\alpha}{2}\right)}\right)^2 \sigma^2}{(N-1)e^2 + \left(Z_{\left(1-\frac{\alpha}{2}\right)}\right)^2 \sigma^2} \tag{3.2}
$$

Where : N is the size of the total population equal to 634, Z is the associated critical coefficient for a confidence level of 95%, α is the significance level equal to 5%, σ is the standard deviation equal to 3 (this value is deduced from a primary study), e is the margin of error equal to 0.5.

From these data, we obtain the following value for the critical coefficient Z :

$$
Z_{1-0.05/2} = Z_{0.975} = 1.96 \tag{3.3}
$$

Hence the value of the sample size n :

$$n = \frac{634(1.96)^2(3)^2}{(633)(0.5)^2 + (1.96)^2(3)^2} \approx 114 \tag{3.4}$$

In the second stage, the questionnaire was distributed to 114 healthcare professionals in the hospital concerned. The schedule adopted for the distribution and collection of the data is shown in the following stages (Boughaba et al. 2019):

- E_1 . Providing information to target professionals to prepare them for the PSC evaluation process and the issues it presents for their establishment;
- E_2 . Distribution of the questionnaire to participants in paper format ;
- E_3 . Letter reminding participants of the value of their involvement in the PSC evaluation exercise. The purpose of this reminder letter is to ensure that participating professionals do not fail to respond;
- E_4 . Retrieving responses and assessing the response rate ;
- E_5 . Thanks and information from participating professionals on the results of the operation (feedback).

If the response rate is insufficient, it will be necessary to return to stage E_3 . It should be noted that stages E_1 , E_2 and E_5 each last one week. Stage E_3 lasts three weeks. Stage E_4 lasts four weeks. The total duration of the PSC evaluation in the pilot hospital was therefore two and a half months.

The data collected was entered into a computer where responses were recorded on a 5-point scale ranging from (5) strongly agree to (1) strongly disagree. Statistic Package for Social Sciences (SPSS) software was used in this study, along with various tests including: descriptive statistical analysis (i.e. frequencies, means and standard deviations), inferential statistics (ANOVA) and reliability analysis (Cronbach Alpha).

In the third stage, the results obtained will be detailed and interpreted in order to identify the problematic dimensions considered to be undeveloped and to propose action plans to improve the institution's PSC. In addition, these results will provide an initial diagnosis of PSC in the Algerian context.

3.2.2. Results

a. Analysis of respondents' socio-demographic characteristics

The socio-demographic characteristics of the study participants (**Table 3.1**) show that the gender ratio is 59% in favour of women. This is due to this component's interest in working in healthcare establishments, confirming the characteristic of the profession. The professionals surveyed are young, with an average age of around 38, and 46% have less than ten years' experience. Most professionals are nurses (34.2%), followed by care assistants (24.6%) and doctors (12.3%). 74.6% of respondents hold permanent positions.

Table 3.1. Socio-demographic characteristics of respondents (Boughaba et al. 2019).

		n	%			n	%
Type	Men	47	41.2	*Years (of age)*	20 - 30	30	26.3
	Women	67	58.8		31 - 40	42	36.8
Seniority (years)	0 - 1	18	15.8		41 - 50	41	36
	2 - 10	52	45.6		≥ 51	1	0.9
	11 - 20	21	18.4			n/N	%
	≥ 20	23	20.2	*Professional category*	Auxiliary nurse	28/156	24.5
Employment contracts	Internal	12	10.5		Nurse	39/217	34.2
	FTC	5	4.4		Doctor	14/78	12.3
	SVP	12	10.5		Administrative Personal	10/55	8.8
	Permanent	85	74.6		Other	23/128	20.2

b. Reliability test (Alpha Cronbach)

The most widely used reliability test for measuring scales is the 'Cronbach Alpha'. This indicator provides information on the homogeneity of the scale and the internal consistency of the linking elements. The higher the internal consistency, approaching a value of 1, the greater the consistency of the responses. The minimum value deemed satisfactory is 0.7 (Cleff 2014; Kottner and Streiner 2010). The results show that the reliability indices are above 0.70 for the 10 survey dimensions, which confirms the validity of the measures (**Table 3.2**).

Table 3.3. Alpha Cronbach reliability scores (Boughaba et al. 2019).

Dimensions	Reliability
	Alpha coefficient
Dim_1 - Overall perceptions of safety	0.88
Dim_2 - Frequency of events reported	0.87
Dim_3 - Supervisor/manager expectations and actions to promote safety	0.79
Dim_4 - Organisational learning and continuous improvement	0.89
Dim_5 - Teamwork on hospital wards	0.80
Sun_6 - Opening of communications	0.76
Dim_7 - Non-punitive response to an error	0.87
Dim_8 - Recruitment	0.74
Dim_9 - Supporting management in ensuring safe care	0.80
Dim_{10} - Teamwork in hospital wards	0.90

c. Overall result

The results of the scores of the ten dimensions are summarized in (**Figure 3.2**) where only three dimensions among the ten dimensions of the CSP selected are above the threshold relative to the developed CSP (Boughaba et al. 2019). These dimensions are Dim_5, Dim_{10}, Dim_1 which successively scored 78.5%, 77.3% and 76.3%. These results confirm that the majority of SSC dimensions are below the 0.75 threshold in the pilot establishment studied. This prompts us to carry out an in-depth analysis of the results obtained in order to improve the diagnosis of PSC in this establishment.

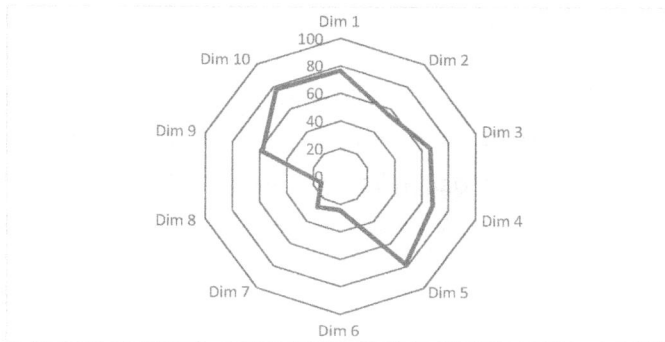

Figure 3.2. UMC level of the establishment studied.

3.2.3. Discussion

In the pilot establishment studied, the perception of PSC is perceived, for the majority of dimensions, as 'underdeveloped'. As a result, and in accordance with the objectives of the NSS, seven dimensions of PSC should be prioritised for development within this hospital. This prioritisation of the development of these dimensions is directly proportional to their scores: $Dim_8 \rightarrow Dim_6 \rightarrow Dim_7 \rightarrow Dim_2 \rightarrow Dim_9 \rightarrow Dim_3 \rightarrow Dim_4$.

The development of these seven dimensions should not lead us to forget the continuous improvement of the three dimensions (Dim_5, Dim_{10} and Dim_1) whose scores exceeded 75%. In addition to information on the scores of the seven problematic dimensions of the PSC of this pilot hospital, the present study sheds light on certain secondary information associated with the scores obtained.

To illustrate our point, we would point out that the evaluation of the "Staffing" dimension raises the problem of staff shortages to cope with the workload, with respondents confirming that this situation means that staff at this pilot hospital work more hours than recommended for patient care. This has a direct impact on the quality and safety of care. This problem is exacerbated during on-call periods, when the situation is problematic in most Algerian health establishments (Heroual et al. 2016).

With regard to "Communication openness", respondents gave negative answers (Strongly Disagree or Disagree) to all three items in this dimension. These results highlight a rigid relational atmosphere between hospital staff and their managers. The result is a passive attitude towards the reporting of adverse events.

However, the development of this dimension is only possible through open communication, as confirmed by a large number of authors (Pattison and Kline 2015; Rabbani et al. 2009). Consequently, the introduction of open communication should be clearly recommended in the SNS.

The same observation was made for the "Non-punitive response to error" dimension, where the results once again confirmed the presence of a rigid relational atmosphere which constitutes an obstacle to the development of PSC. In this context, it has been shown that among the obstacles encountered in reporting errors are a lack of confidentiality, follow-up and fear of repercussions (McArdle, Burns, and Ireland 2003; Moumtzoglou 2010; Pattison and Kline 2015).

It would therefore be necessary to establish a PSC environment in which adverse events can be reported without individuals being identified, giving staff the opportunity to learn from their mistakes and, where possible, make improvements to prevent future human and technical errors, thereby promoting safe care (Pattison and Kline 2015). To develop this dimension, we propose incorporating into the SNS the experience gained in other sectors, such as the procedure that has enhanced the reporting of adverse events in the Algerian petrochemicals sector, based on the Stop-Card procedure procedure (Mouda et al. 2016).

In addition, it is important to remember that this first study on the evaluation of UMC in a pilot hospital establishment enabled us, on the one hand, to have a snapshot of the level of UMC in this establishment and, on the other hand, to identify possible perspectives for the follow-up to be given to this study. In particular, the evaluation of UMC should be carried out in the context of a national project to promote UMC.

It is in the context of such a project that the methodology adopted in this study is to be used in a number of hospitals with the aim of making comparisons between them in terms of PSC and proposing action plans to improve PSC in the NHS.

The reason for considering such a project is that, often, PSC evaluations are carried out in isolation and informally. This makes it less likely that follow-up action will be taken. However, if the evaluation of CSP is overseen by a national project such as the Algerian CSP observatory, the evaluation and improvement of CSP will be formalised and carried out in a coherent and concise manner; this will give it greater legitimacy and greater involvement on the part of health establishments.

In this context, we present our second contribution, which aims to evaluate PSC using the dimensional approach as part of a national observatory project dedicated to PSC.

3.3. Evaluation of CSP as part of the Algerian CS observatory project P

First of all, the aim of this second contribution is twofold: to highlight, in the short term, the following two key facts: (i) the problematic dimensions of the hospitals studied, and (ii) the possibility of classifying these hospitals according to their respective levels of PSC.

In the medium term, the rankings awarded to the hospitals studied as part of the national PSC observatory (ASCO) project will encourage the lower-ranked hospitals to improve their rankings and, as a result, improve the level of PSC at national level (i.e. within the framework of the NHS).

3.3.1. Materials & Methods

a. Study design, parameters and participants

In order to initiate the ASCO project, a cross-sectional multicentre study was conducted over the period from 2018 to 2019, which included 10 Algerian public health establishments (EHs). The EHs concerned were contacted before the start of the study to obtain their approvals, where it was explained that their participation is not mandatory, but it is strongly recommended to evaluate the PSC. In addition, it was explained that the results obtained will enable their establishments to be ranked in relation to other organisations in the same sector, and will serve as a snapshot to monitor future developments in PSC (Fourar et al. 2020).

After obtaining their agreement, an initial census was carried out of the professionals (n = 4360) working in the healthcare establishments studied (EH). The questionnaire was distributed to participants (*n = 1370*) using convenience sampling in which all professional categories were included (i.e. doctors, nurses, administrators, etc.). A timetable for distributing and collecting the questionnaire was drawn up. This schedule consisted of 4 stages and was spread over a minimum period of two months for each EH in order to achieve a satisfactory response rate:

- E_1 . Inform targeted professionals about the PSC assessment by distributing letters of explanation;

- E$_2$. Distribution of the questionnaire to targeted professionals in paper format ;
- E$_3$. Retrieving responses and assessing the response rate ;
- E$_4$. Acknowledge respondents' participation and share feedback.

b. Choice of study instrument

The selection of a single instrument for measuring PSC helps to ensure the success of the ASCO project. For this purpose, we chose the HSOPSC questionnaire, the reasons for which were presented at the beginning of this chapter.

c. Data analysis

The "Statistical Package for the Social Sciences (SPSS) version 20" software was used in this study, along with various tests including descriptive statistical analysis (i.e. frequency, mean, standard deviation, percentage) and reliability analysis. In this respect, the most common reliability test for scale measures is the "Cronbach Alpha". This indicator provides information on the homogeneity of the scale and the internal consistency of the connecting elements. The higher the internal consistency (i.e. approaching a value of 1), the more elements contribute to the construction. The minimum value deemed satisfactory is 0.7 (Cleff 2014; Kottner and Streiner 2010).. In addition, the difference in significance between the dimensions of UMC and various socio-demographic and occupational variables was estimated using inferential statistics (ANOVA). The significance level was set at 0.05.

The dimensional scores were calculated for the study sample as a whole, and then for each PE using Eq (3.5) :

$$S_{D_i} = \frac{np_i}{N_i} \; ; i = 1...10 \qquad\qquad (3.5)$$

With : S_{D_i} being the score for the i dimension of SC, np_i is the number of positive responses for this i dimension and N_i is the total number of responses for this i dimension, including positive, negative and neutral responses.

The dimensions are then assessed according to their scores, where a dimension is said to be developed if it had a score of 75% or more. If the dimension had a score of 50% or less, the dimension is said to be undeveloped. Dimensions with scores between 50% and 75% are considered underdeveloped (Reis et al. 2018).

d. EHs classification

The aim of the ASCO project, once the PSC has been assessed, is to rank the HEIs according to their PSC profile. This classification is based on the descending order of the number of dimensions developed. For those HEs that share the same number of developed dimensions, they are classified in descending order of underdeveloped dimensions. Lastly, the HEs that share the same number of underdeveloped dimensions are classified using the descending order of undeveloped dimensions.

3.3.2. Results

a. Characteristics of the target sample

A total of 1118 professionals responded to the questionnaire. During statistical processing, 168 questionnaires were rejected due to non-compliant responses. As a result, 950 questionnaires were retained for this study, representing a response rate of 69% of the sample size (n = 1370) and 30% of the total workforce (n = 4136). These percentages are considered more than sufficient to validate the results of the study given that a number of authors recommend using a sample size that represents 10% of the total population to study a phenomenon (Cleff 2014).

The response rate based on professional category in terms of sample size ranged from 6.7% to 51.1%. Nurses had the highest representation (51.1%), followed by physicians (30.2%). Administrators and other categories had the lowest representation in the sample, with response rates of 6.7% and 12% respectively (**Table 3.3**). In terms of seniority, 16.3% had less than 2 years' work experience, 26.5% between 2 and 10 years, 35% between 11 and 20 years, and 22.2% more than 20 years.

Table 3.3. Socio-demographic characteristics of respondents (Fourar et al. 2020).

Characteristics	Frequency (n)	Percentage (%)
Total	950	100
Gender		
Man	396	41,7
Woman	554	58,3
Seniority (years)		
0–01	155	16.3
2–10	252	26.5
11–20	332	35
⩾20	211	22.2
Work contract		
Intern	141	14.8
FDC	146	15.4
UDC	215	22.6
Permanent	448	47.2
Age (years)		
20–30	255	26.9
31–40	237	24.9
41–50	248	26.1
⩾51	210	22.1
Professional category		
Nurse	485	51,1
Doctor	287	30,2
Administrative staff	64	6,7
Other	114	12

b. Reliability test

To check the reliability of the questionnaire, Cronbach's alpha test was calculated. The alpha values for all dimensions ranged from 0.70 to 0.88 (**Table**

3.4), which confirmed that the reliability of the scale measurement was satisfactory in this study.

c. Scores for dimensions of CSP

The scores for the PSC dimensions were calculated globally for the study sample (**Table 3.4**). They were then calculated for each of the 10 EHs (**Table 3.5**) as explained previously (see Materials & Method). They were also represented in the form of radar graphs (Appendix 2). All the dimensions that obtained a score of less than 50% are considered to be undeveloped, and are therefore problematic for the PSC.

Table 3.4. Positive response rates and Cronbach's α reliability scores. (Fourar et al. 2020).

Dimensions	Positive responses (%)	Alpha coefficient
D1 - Overall perceptions of safety	56.7	0.85
D2 - Frequency of events reported	62	0.84
D3 - Supervisor/manager expectations and actions to promote safety	50	0.82
D4 - Organisational learning - continuous improvement	61.6	0.83
D5 - Teamwork within hospital units	64	0.86
D6 - Opening communications	41.7	0.70
D7 - Non-punitive response to an error	31.9	0.78
D8 - Recruitment	26	0.76
D9 - Supporting management in ensuring safe care	37	0.85
D10 - Teamwork on hospital wards	39.5	0.88

Table 3.5. HE dimensional scores (Fourar et al. 2020).

	D_1	D_2	D_3	D_4	D_5	D_6	D_7	D_8	D_9	D_{10}
HE_1	50.3	57.4	63.9	70.9	74.8	66.1	41.6	38.7	32.2	37.7
HE_2	76.3	56.1	66.4	68.1	78.5	24.3	27.2	14.3	57.9	77.3
HE_3	65.9	44.8	48.7	54.1	69.4	28.7	35.1	24.7	53.4	50.9
HE_4	56	62.5	66.8	70.2	78.4	55.8	30.8	42.9	33.7	38.1
HE_5	51.4	62	50.7	58.9	68.1	47.2	28.7	40.7	37	41.2
HE_6	70.1	60.8	63.7	66.3	76.5	33.7	31.7	20.9	63.1	76.6
HE_7	42.2	52.1	59.5	65.1	70.4	55.9	39.5	29.9	33.7	44.1
HE_8	50.6	48.4	50	57.7	64	41.1	34.1	26	38.8	42.1
HE_9	33.2	28.3	31.3	36.1	48.6	23.2	14.9	14.1	27.2	35
HE_{10}	71.4	66.7	57.1	68.6	76.8	40.5	35.7	26.2	52.4	44

a. Associated variables of CSP

In order to estimate the significant differences between the dimensions of the CSP and the characteristics of the sample, the one-factor ANOVA test was applied. Frequencies, mean scores and standard deviations were also calculated for the set of variables (i.e. gender, age, seniority, type of contract, professional category) (**Table 3.6**).

Table 3.6. One-way ANOVA Test values (Fourar et al. 2020).

Characteristic	N	D_1 Mean ± SD	D_2 Mean ± SD	D_3 Mean ± SD	D_4 Mean ± SD	D_5 Mean ± SD	D_6 Mean ± SD	D_7 Mean ± SD	D_8 Mean ± SD	D_9 Mean ± SD	D_{10} Mean ± SD
Gender											
Man	396	3.69 ± 1.04	3.61 ± 0.79	3.73 ± 0.80	3.71 ± 0.71	3.79 ± 1.75	3.51 ± 1.25	2.64 ± 0.72	2.58 ± 0.77	2.95 ± 1.20	2.98 ± 1.21
Woman	554	3.62 ± 0.95	3.54 ± 1.06	3.68 ± 0.98	3.64 ± 1.23	3.61 ± 1.93	3.44 ± 1.23	2.71 ± 1.01	2.65 ± 1.09	3.04 ± 0.68	3.02 ± 1.19
		$P = 0.282$	$P = 0.226$	$P = 0.403$	$P = 0.309$	$P = 0.878$	$P = 0.390$	$P = 0.237$	$P = 0.272$	$P = 0.142$	$P = 0.612$
Age											
20–30	255	3.21 ± 0.51	3.05 ± 1.01	3.42 ± 1.08	3.51 ± 0.94	3.69 ± 1.53	3.56 ± 1.06	2.49 ± 0.48	2.25 ± 0.32	3.49 ± 0.87	3.51 ± 0.92
31–40	237	3.27 ± 0.93	3.29 ± 0.82	3.73 ± 0.85	3.69 ± 0.83	3.79 ± 0.80	3.67 ± 1.14	2.55 ± 0.97	2.49 ± 0.91	3.52 ± 0.54	3.62 ± 1.10
41–50	248	3.34 ± 0.74	3.12 ± 1.04	3.65 ± 0.84	3.66 ± 0.85	3.71 ± 0.79	3.59 ± 1.10	2.52 ± 0.91	2.46 ± 0.85	3.48 ± 1.26	3.53 ± 1.06
>51	210	3.32 ± 0.52	3.24 ± 0.59	3.91 ± 0.69	3.78 ± 0.73	3.52 ± 1.04	3.69 ± 1.40	2.67 ± 1.21	2.51 ± 1.15	3.65 ± 0.46	3.83 ± 1.36
		$P = 0.165$	$P = 0.012$	$P = 0.075$	$P = 0.0061$	$P = 0.068$	$P = 0.573$	$P = 0.174$	$P = 0.002$	$P = 0.137$	$P = 0.009$
Seniority											
0–01	155	3.49 ± 1.03	3.69 ± 1.10	3.58 ± 0.81	3.59 ± 1.10	3.19 ± 0.86	3.48 ± 1.06	2.57 ± 1.30	2.51 ± 1.24	3.37 ± 0.77	3.14 ± 1.02
2–10	252	3.81 ± 1.14	3.71 ± 0.94	3.73 ± 0.85	3.71 ± 0.94	3.28 ± 0.90	3.55 ± 1.05	2.85 ± 1.07	2.79 ± 1.01	3.44 ± 0.81	3.21 ± 1.01
11–20	332	3.52 ± 1.21	3.67 ± 0.85	3.70 ± 0.69	3.67 ± 0.85	3.36 ± 0.74	3.42 ± 1.28	2.44 ± 0.72	2.38 ± 0.66	3.31 ± 0.65	3.28 ± 1.24
>20	211	3.48 ± 1.11	3.72 ± 0.80	3.67 ± 0.73	3.72 ± 0.80	3.23 ± 0.78	3.31 ± 0.98	2.61 ± 0.95	2.55 ± 0.89	3.39 ± 0.69	3.07 ± 0.94
		$P = 0.003$	$P = 0.922$	$P = 0.262$	$P = 0.004$	$P = 0.117$	$P = 0.008$	$P = 0.002$	$P = 0.055$	$P = 0.188$	$P = 0.012$
Work contract											
Intern	141	1.80 ± 0.53	1.70 ± 0.91	2.55 ± 0.58	1.70 ± 0.44	2.61 ± 0.53	3.28 ± 0.75	2.08 ± 1.03	1.51 ± 0.21	2.78 ± 0.49	2.94 ± 0.71
FDC	146	1.76 ± 0.44	2.53 ± 0.56	2.75 ± 0.39	2.53 ± 0.56	2.81 ± 1.34	3.30 ± 1.30	2.01 ± 0.99	1.94 ± 0.14	3.10 ± 1.30	3.26 ± 1.26
UDC	215	2.15 ± 0.46	3.40 ± 1.06	3.31 ± 0.89	3.40 ± 0.64	3.37 ± 0.84	3.38 ± 1.10	2.33 ± 0.52	2.37 ± 0.84	3.22 ± 0.79	3.48 ± 1.06
Permanent	448	3.21 ± 0.83	3.54 ± 1.03	3.89 ± 0.45	3.99 ± 0.60	4.14 ± 1.21	3.45 ± 0.93	2.41 ± 0.82	2.85 ± 0.95	3.32 ± 1.23	3.58 ± 0.97
		$P = 0.000$	$P = 0.000$	$P = 0.000$	$P = 0.000$	$P = 0.000$	$P = 0.222$	$P = 0.000$	$P = 0.000$	$P = 0.000$	$P = 0.000$
Prof. Category											
Nurse	485	3.81 ± 0.83	3.56 ± 0.78	3.61 ± 0.69	3.47 ± 0.74	3.67 ± 0.64	3.49 ± 1.27	2.67 ± 0.70	2.61 ± 1.07	3.39 ± 0.61	3.44 ± 1.23
Doctor	287	3.57 ± 0.53	4.07 ± 0.50	4.15 ± 0.34	4.09 ± 0.48	3.98 ± 0.29	3.62 ± 0.93	3.86 ± 0.35	3.80 ± 0.76	3.47 ± 1.26	3.52 ± 0.89
Administrator	64	3.24 ± 1.13	3.64 ± 0.69	3.68 ± 0.75	3.70 ± 0.79	3.74 ± 0.71	3.23 ± 1.25	2.70 ± 0.75	2.64 ± 0.58	3.24 ± 0.72	3.19 ± 1.21
Other	114	2.68 ± 1.19	3.05 ± 0.86	3.06 ± 1.06	3.20 ± 1.19	3.12 ± 1.01	3.41 ± 0.67	2.18 ± 1.06	2.45 ± 1.45	3.41 ± 1.17	3.45 ± 1.71
		$P = 0.000$	$P = 0.000$	$P = 0.000$	$P = 0.000$	$P = 0.000$	$P = 0.052$	$P = 0.000$	$P = 0.011$	$P = 0.319$	$P = 0.272$

b. EHs classification

The results in **Table 3.5** are used as a basis for classifying HE according to the three PSC ordered dimensional criteria (**Table 3.7**). As part of the ASCO project, this classification is capitalised in the form of radar graphs (see Appendix 2).

Table 3.7. Classification of WSS in the ASCO project project (Fourar et al. 2020).

Rank	HE_i	Type of HE	R.R (%)	Criteria 1 Nb. D_i	Criteria 1 D_i array	Criteria 2 Nb. D_i	Criteria 2 D_i array	Criteria 3 Nb. D_i	Criteria 3 D_i array	Detailed results as a Radar graph
1	HE_2	HC	18	3	[76.3 – 78.5]	4	[56.1 – 68.1]	3	[14.3 – 17.2]	
2	HE_6	SHC	23.3	2	[76.5 – 76.6]	5	[60.9 – 70.1]	3	[20.9 – 33.7]	
3	HE_4	SHC	60.1	1	[78.4]	5	[55.8 – 70.2]	4	[30.8 – 42.9]	
4	HE_{10}	EBC	25.9	1	[76.8]	5	[52.4 – 71.4]	4	[26.2 – 44]	Cf. Annex 2
5	HE_1	UHC	16.4			6	[50.3 – 74.8]	4	[32.2 – 41.6]	
6	HE_7	SHC	24.8			5	[52.1 – 70.4]	5	[29.9 – 44.1]	
7	HE_3	HC	32.2			5	[50.9 – 69.4]	5	[24.7 – 48.7]	
8	HE_5	SHC	14			5	[50.7 – 68.1]	5	[28.7 – 47.2]	
9	HE_8	EBS	35.5			4	[50 - 64]	6	[26 – 48.4]	
10	HE_9	EBC	25.9					10	[14.1 48.6]	

UHC = University Hospital Center; HC = Hospital Center; EBC = Establishment of Basic Care; SHC = Specialized Hospital Center;
R.R = Response rate;
Criteria 1. Developed dimensions; Criteria 2. Underdeveloped dimensions; Criteria 3. Non-developed dimensions

3.3.3. Discussion

This study was carried out to evaluate the PSC in Algerian hospitals as part of the first national federative project called "Algerian Safety Culture Observatory - ASCO-", which enables hospitals to be involved in a voluntary but dynamic way in the new reforms of the NHS. The high response rate of 69% testifies to the involvement of healthcare professionals in this initiative. It should be noted that similar response rates have been reported in several studies and have been deemed satisfactory (Boughaba et al. 2019; Chen et al. 2019; Occelli et al. 2013; Özcan, Kaya, and Teleş 2020; Tlili et al. 2020).

a. Dimensions of the CS P

In HEIs, PSC is perceived as underdeveloped. All the dimensions therefore need to be the subject of a holistic promotion strategy. The dimensions that were not developed were 'Non-punitive response to error', 'Staffing', 'Communication openness', 'Management support for care safety' and 'Teamwork across hospital units', with scores of 31.9%, 26%, 41.7%, 37% and 39.5% respectively. These dimensions should therefore be prioritised in the proposed promotion strategy because of their crucial importance in improving patient safety.

For example, insufficient staff to manage the workload has a direct impact on the occurrence of AEs and consequently on patient safety (Sabry et al. 2020). In terms of 'Communication openness', 'Management support for care safety' & 'Teamwork across hospital units', respondents gave negative answers on these three dimensions, which are considered essential for reducing the occurrence of adverse events.

As a result, the SNS is characterised by a blame culture where professionals are punished for their mistakes. These results are in line with the findings of the first study that was conducted to evaluate PSC in a pilot Algerian hospital, where the same problematic dimensions were identified (Boughaba et al. 2019).

In another study, the two dimensions 'Staffing' and 'Non-punitive response to error' were found to be problematic for US hospitals (Famolaro et al. 2018). To remedy this, a just participatory culture based on open communication and a non-punitive response to error needs to be adapted as confirmed by a number of authors (Boughaba et al. 2019; Goh et al. 2013).

The underdeveloped dimensions 'Overall perceptions of safety', 'Frequency of events reported', 'Supervisor/manager's expectations and actions promoting safety', 'Organizational learning-continuous improvement' and 'Teamwork within hospital units' need to be integrated into a holistic approach aimed at improving patient safety within the NHS.

b. Variables associated with CS P

Analysis of the means of the SSC dimensions by son-in-law shows that the scores vary between the female and male sons-in-law, while the ANOVA test showed no significance. For the age variable, mean scores showed differences between age groups, statistical significance was found for the dimensions 'Frequency of events reported', 'Organizational learning-Continuous improvement', 'Staffing' & 'Teamwork across hospital units' with p-values of 0.012, 0.0061, 0.002 and 0.009 respectively. The lowest mean scores were identified for the age group (20-30 years) for most dimensions.

The analysis of variance for the seniority variable shows statistical significance for the dimensions 'Overall perception of safety', 'Organizational learning-continuous improvement', 'Teamwork across hospital units', 'communication openness' & 'Non-punitive response to error'. For the professional category, the analysis of variance shows statistical significance for all dimensions, with the exception of 'communication openness'.

Analysis of the average scores shows that the highest values were found in the group of doctors. For the category of employment contracts, the highest mean scores were found for permanent employees, followed by permanent contracts (UTC). Statistical significance was found for all dimensions except two, which were 'Management support for patient safety' & 'Teamwork across hospital units'.

These results show that the variables 'length of service', 'employment contract' and 'occupational category' have an impact on the dimensions of PSC. The same conclusions were reached by (Boughaba et al. 2019)where it was found that the variables 'employment contract' and 'occupational categories' have a direct impact on PSC. For (Tlili et al. 2020)the seniority and occupational category variables had a significant impact on the dimensions of PSC in Tunisia, while the type of contract was not included in their study.

c. EHs classification

The ranking of the HEIs (**Table 3.7**) shows that the first four establishments share practically the same level of maturity of the PSC, where the dimensions considered as 'developed' and 'underdeveloped' are in the majority compared with the 'undeveloped'. The hospitals ranked from 5 to 8 share virtually the same level of PSC maturity, with 'underdeveloped' dimensions dominating over those of the 'underdeveloped' type. The lowest maturity levels are those of EH_9 and EH_{10} where the 'Undeveloped' dimensions are dominant for EH_9 and systematic for EH_{10}. For these two EHs, it is necessary to categorically review the health policy within their structures in order to promote their CSP. The advantage of classifying HEIs as part of the ASCO project is that it enables classified HEIs to make greater efforts to consolidate their position.

In this way, the ASCO project will provide a real barometer for the dynamic evaluation of PSC within the Algerian NHS. Better still, the ASCO project will serve as a motivational tool for Algerian healthcare institutions to join the initiative to improve PSC. Consequently, the monitoring of PSC indicators over time and the generalisation of the assessment of the level of maturity of the PSC of other Algerian EHs will make it possible to promote patient safety in the SNS.

d. Limits of the study

The sample for this study was limited to just 10 Algerian hospitals in order to launch the ASCO project. Therefore, a more representative sample needs to be studied in order to be able to generalise the results to the entire Algerian NHS. In addition, a longitudinal study is recommended in order to monitor the evolution of PSC over time and provide a dynamic classification of the EHs.

3.4. Conclusion

Throughout this chapter, we have focused on the assessment of PSC using the HSOPSC questionnaire in order to describe healthcare professionals' perceptions of safety in a health care organisation. In the first study, relating to a pilot healthcare establishment, the assessment of PSC gave us a snapshot of the level of PSC, where the dimensions 'Staffing', 'Communication openness' and 'Non-punitive response to error' were considered problematic and in need of strengthening. This study encouraged us to extend it to a set of EHs covered by the ASCO project.

This gradual generalisation of the evaluation of PSC in Algerian Hospitals will undoubtedly make it possible to draw up joint action plans to establish PSC at national level. In line with the results obtained, the priority areas for improvement in the SNS are: 'Staffing', 'Communication openness', 'Non-punitive response to error' and 'Management support for care Safety'. In addition, the second study drew our attention to the importance of mixed evaluations of PSC (qualitative-quantitative evaluation), which is also recommended by certain authors (Guldenmund 2010; Occelli 2018; Reis et al. 2018).

Chapter IV

The contribution of Maturity Models to the study of PSC

4.1. Introduction

In the previous chapter, the focus was on the promotion of PHC in the Algerian context. Our two contributions in the previous chapter confirmed that the evaluation of PSC should be a priority for health organisations. As a reminder, this evaluation of CSP was carried out using the dimensional approach. The literature specialising in PSC states that this approach suffers from a number of limitations. (Cooper 2016; Fleming 2007; Guldenmund 2010; Hodgen et al. 2017) :

- Dimensional assessments are reduced to measuring individual attitudes and practices in a "*safety climate*" context;
- Beyond the use of the HSOPSC questionnaire alone, the wide variation in the dimensions explored and their items makes comparative studies inappropriate;
- There is a problem of aggregating the CSP dimensional scores in order to calculate its overall score.

This last constraint drew our attention and enabled us to pose two new scientific research questions relating to PSC:

Q_1 - *If it is difficult to aggregate all the dimensions of the PSC, is it possible to settle for a partial aggregation of these dimensions?*

Q_2 - *If so, is it possible to capitalise on this partial aggregation for the purposes of a mixed evaluation of the PSC (qualitative-quantitative evaluation)?*

The aim of this final chapter is to provide some answers to these two questions. Our answers will undoubtedly lead to the development of a mixed approach to the evaluation of PSC (i.e. the combined use of dimensional and typological approaches to the evaluation of PSC).

In the context of this merging of the two approaches to assessing PSC, it is important to remember that several authors advocate the use of a combined method of assessing PSC (i.e. Quantitative and Qualitative) rather than simply relying on a single approach (Ginsburg et al. 2009; Halligan and Zecevic 2011; Pumar-Méndez, Attree, and Wakefield 2014). However, this new mixed approach has only recently been adopted (Granel et al. 2020).

For example, (Listyowardojo et al. 2017) assessed PSC in a Chinese healthcare facility using the Safety Attitude Questionnaire (SAQ) followed by staff interviews. Similarly, (Roney et al. 2017) used a questionnaire to assess nurses' concerns about patient safety in the US, followed by focus groups to discuss their expectations. In another study, (Granel et al. 2020) conducted an assessment of PSC in two Spanish public hospitals using the HSOPSC questionnaire accompanied by in-depth interviews and observations.

In our case, we propose to use PCA and K-means methods as support tools for this mixed evaluation of the PSC. This will be the subject of the next section.

4.2. Contribution of PCA/K-means to the mixed evaluation of CS P

4.2.1. Materials & Methods

It should be noted that our contribution consists of a proposal for a mixed evaluation of the PSC in a set of hospital establishments. These are the establishments selected in the last part of the previous chapter. Initially, PSC is assessed quantitatively using the HSOPSC questionnaire, in which ten dimensions of PSC are assessed individually. The next step is to attempt to partially group these dimensions using PCA and K-means methods (**Figure 4.1**).

Indeed, in step 1 of Figure 4.1, the application of Principal Component Analysis (PCA) aims to visualise the dimensions of the PSC in a space formed by a minimum of principal components, which are generally two in number (Hefaidh and Mébarek, 2020) which help to preserve as many linear links as possible between these dimensions, and therefore to identify their potential grouping.

As a reminder, PCA is one of the most widely used methods for reducing the dimensionality of data while retaining important information (Hadef and Djebabra 2019a; Karamizadeh et al. 2013; Palese 2018). It allows existing similarities between individuals to be identified. These similarities are explained by the notion of linear link or correlation coefficient between the variables. These variables are then combined into a smaller set of uncorrelated artificial variables called principal components (Shirali, Shekari and Angali, 2016). This combination is defined so that the first principal component represents the greatest possible variability.

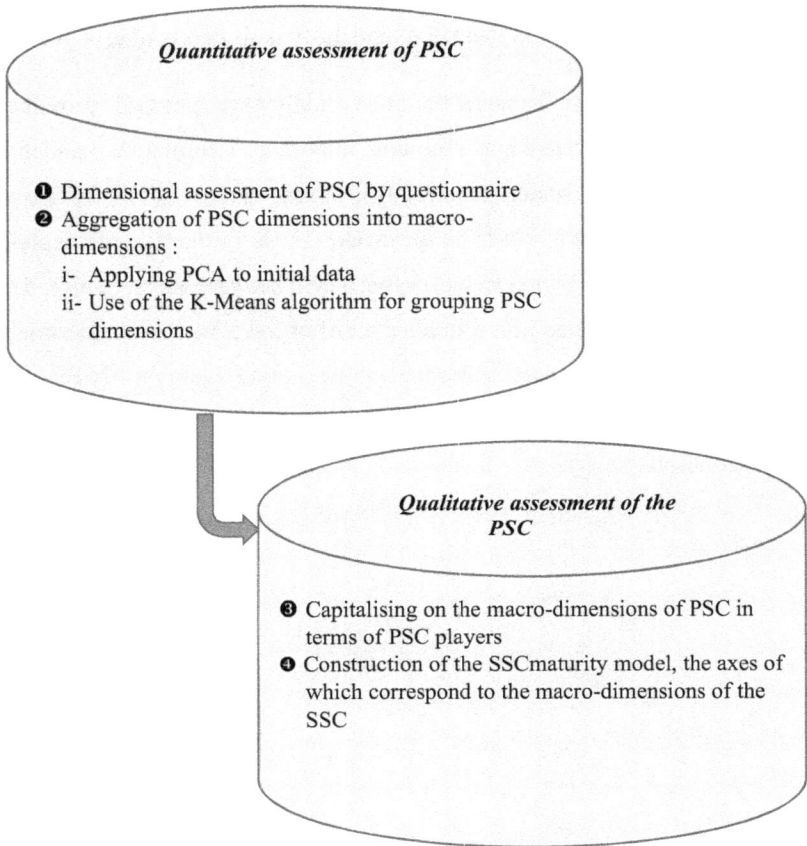

Figure 4.1. Steps in the proposed method for the mixed assessment of PSC.

To illustrate, we assume the existence of m variables (Dimension Scores) and n individuals (SSC Dimensions) and consider the $n \times m$ data matrix: $D = (d_1, d_2,..., d_m)$ where each row represents the values of each variable for each dimension.

The CPA application process can be summarised as follows (Hadef and Djebabra 2019b) :

- Preparing data in matrix form ;
- Calculating the correlation matrix ;
- Calculation of eigenvalues and eigenvectors ;
- Calculation of the coordinates of the dimensions (of the CS in our case) ;
- Representation of the dimensions of the PSC in space (F1, F2).

To ensure the statistical validity of the results, the sample must be relatively large. However, a ratio of ten individuals per variable is considered sufficient to conduct the analysis (Hair et al., 2014).

The second stage involves validating the grouping of the CSP dimensions into distinct groups. To do this, Clustering Analysis provides a better understanding of the data by dividing individuals into groups (Clusters) of individuals, so that individuals in one group are more similar than individuals in other groups (Penkova 2017).

The K-means algorithm is one of the best-known cluster analysis techniques (Fränti and Sieranoja, 2019; Zhu, Idemudia and Feng, 2019).. It is an unsupervised classification algorithm based on a prototype that attempts to find K non-overlapping groups from n individuals. These groups are represented by their prototypes or also known as centroids (a centroid of a group is generally the average of the points of this group). (Fränti and Sieranoja 2019)).

The K-means algorithm can be expressed as an objective function that depends on the proximities of the data points to the centroids of the group, as follows:

$$min_{\{mk\},\ 1<k<K} \sum_{k=1}^{K} \sum_{x \in C_k} \pi_x\ dist\ (x, m_k) \qquad (4.1)$$

Where : π_x is the weight of x, n_k is the number of variables assigned to the group C_k K is the number of clusters defined by the user, and the "$dist$"

function calculates the distance between individual x and the centroid m_k, $1 < k < K$.

In equation (1), m_k is expressed as :

$$m_k = \sum_{x \in c_k} \frac{\pi_x x}{n_k} \qquad (4.2)$$

It is common for PCA to be used to project individuals into a low-dimensional subspace and for K-means then to be applied in subspace (Ding and He, 2004; Zhu, Idemudia and Feng, 2019). Therefore, the K-means algorithm follows the following steps:

- Preparation of data in matrix form (supplied by the PCA) ;
- Randomly select the initial centroids ;
- Assign individuals to the nearest centroid ;
- Recalculate the centre of each group and modify the centroid;
- Iteration until convergence.

The final results of the K-means algorithm allow us to define the number K of groups of individuals G = $\{G_1, G_2, \ldots\ldots, G_k\}$. These groups are subsequently capitalised to define the groups of dimensions (macro-dimension) of the CSP, where the dimensions of each group share the same properties.

It should be noted that according to the groups obtained from the PCA/K-means approach, the score for each group of dimensions is calculated according to the following formula:

$$S_{G_i} = \frac{\sum_{i=1}^{n} S_{D_i}}{N} \qquad (4.3)$$

Where : S_{G_i} being the global score of the i group, S_{D_i} the score of the i dimension of the CS belonging to the i group and N the number of dimensions in the i group.

These scores are represented on a scale ranging from 'not developed' to 'developed'. As a result, problematic macro-dimensions (score <50%) requiring priority improvement actions can be identified.

Furthermore, the combination of the three possible levels (i.e. ND, UD and D) results in the proposal of a PSC maturity matrix (Figure 4.2). In this respect, the levels "ND and UD" and "UD and D" are considered as adjacent levels, while the levels "ND and D" are not adjacent. This will help define the levels in the maturity matrix. A level is defined when two adjacent levels are combined, keeping the lower value (e.g. ND and UD). In the case of two non-adjacent levels, an intermediate value is retained (e.g. D).

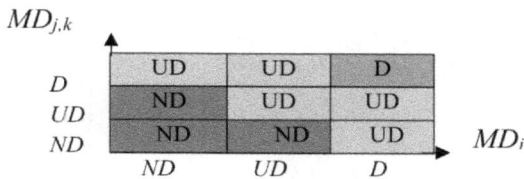

$MD_{j,k}$

	ND	UD	D
D	UD	UD	D
UD	ND	UD	UD
ND	ND	ND	UD

MD_i

Figure 4.2: Proposed PSC matrix.

In addition, it is possible to calculate the surface areas of different zones associated with maturity levels: $S_{ND} = 3/9$; $S_{UD} = 5/9$ & $S_D = 1/9$. By normalising them on a scale of [0-1], we can obtain quantitative scores for the maturity levels:

- $0 < CSP_{ND} \ \square \ 0.33$;

- $0.33 < CSP_{UD} \ \square \ 0.8$;

- $0.89 < CSP_D \ \square \ 1$.

4.2.2. Results

a. Sample, parameters and data collection

As a reminder, the sample selected is that already detailed in the last part of the previous chapter. It consists of a sample of 10 hospitals which have certain characteristics in common, such as staff numbers (mean = 412) and bed capacity (mean = 87), and are made up of similar units such as general surgery, internal medicine, paediatric units and emergency departments. These establishments were part of a pilot study aimed at setting up an Algerian observatory of CSP (see Chapter 3).

To illustrate the interest of the approach proposed in this chapter, the SSC dimensions (*Dim*) are considered as individuals and their scores in the ten hospitals (*EH*) are variables (**Table 4.1**).

Table 4.1. Rate of positive responses for each PSC dimension.

	EH 1	EH 2	EH 3	EH 4	EH 5	EH 6	EH 7	EH 8	EH 9	EH 10
Dim 1	50,3	76,3	65,9	56	51,4	70,1	42,2	50,6	33,2	71,4
Dim 2	57,4	56,1	44,8	62,5	62	60,8	52,1	48,4	28,3	66,7
Dim 3	63,9	66,4	48,7	66,8	50,7	63,7	59,5	50	31,3	57,1
Dim 4	70,9	68,1	54,1	70,2	58,9	66,3	65,1	57,7	36,1	68,6
Dim 5	74,8	78,5	69,4	78,4	68,1	76,5	70,4	64	48,6	76,8
Dim 6	66,1	24,3	28,7	55,8	47,2	33,7	55,9	41,1	23,2	40,5
Sun 7	41,6	27,2	35,1	30,8	28,7	31,7	39,5	34,1	14,9	35,7
Sun 8	38,7	14,3	24,7	42,9	40,7	20,9	29,9	26	14,1	26,2
Sun 9	32,2	57,9	53,4	33,7	37	63,1	33,7	38,8	27,2	52,4
Sun 10	37,7	77,3	50,9	38,1	41,2	76,6	44,1	42,1	35	44

(Dim 1) Overall perceptions of patient safety; (Dim 2) Frequency of reporting adverse events; (Dim 3) Supervisor/manager expectations and actions promoting safety; (Dim 4) Organizational learning-continuous improvement; (Dim 5) Teamwork within units; (Dim 6) Communication openness; (Dim 7) Non-punitive response to error; (Dim 8) Staffing; (Dim 9) Management support for patient safety; (Dim 10) Teamwork across hospital units

b. Application of PCA & K-means

Firstly, the application of PCA requires the calculation of the correlation matrix (**Table 4.2**). Table 4.2 shows that the correlation coefficients calculated between the variables are positively correlated (correlation coefficient varies from 0 to 1). The majority of variables are highly correlated (correlation coefficient > 0.5) with the exception of two cases ('EH 1 and EH 2' = 0.276; 'EH1 and EH 3' = 0.293).

Secondly, the eigenvalues and eigenvectors are calculated in order to identify two principal components which will be used to represent the initial data (**Table**

4.3). In this respect, analysis of the values represented in Table 4.3 shows that the eigenvalue of F1 is equal to 7.528 and the total variability is retained at 75.3% if the variables are represented on the F1 axis. For the F2 axis, we see that the eigenvalue is equal to 1.862 and the total variability is preserved at 18.6%. For the other axes, F3, F4, F5, F6, F7, F8 and F9, variability is preserved at 6.1%. Consequently, the first two principal components are used for the rest of the application given that the variability is preserved at 93.8%.

Table 4.2: Correlation matrix.

	EH 1	EH 2	EH 3	EH 4	EH 5	EH 6	EH 7	EH 8	EH 9	EH 10
EH 1	1									
EH 2	0,276	1								
EH 3	0,293	0,928	1							
EH 4	0,931	0,454	0,462	1						
EH 5	0,812	0,538	0,543	0,941	1					
EH 6	0,261	0,991	0,909	0,432	0,541	1				
EH 7	0,947	0,469	0,431	0,884	0,793	0,469	1			
EH 8	0,785	0,788	0,806	0,847	0,848	0,777	0,868	1		
EH 9	0,570	0,889	0,876	0,691	0,752	0,893	0,722	0,914	1	
EH 10	0,605	0,810	0,870	0,747	0,816	0,802	0,659	0,930	0,837	1

Table 4.3. Eigenvalues obtained by PCA.

	F1	F2	F3	F4	F5	F6	F7	F8	F9
Eigenvalue	7,528	1,862	0,301	0,167	0,085	0,046	0,006	0,005	0,001
Variability (%)	75,279	18,620	3,009	1,668	0,849	0,460	0,061	0,048	0,006
Cumulative	75,279	93,899	96,908	98,576	99,425	99,885	99,946	99,994	100,000

After calculating the coordinates of the dimensions in relation to F1 and F2 (**Table 4.4**), they are represented graphically (see **Figure 4.4**) **in order to** identify potential groupings of the PSC dimensions. However, in our case, the groups cannot be identified. It is therefore necessary to use the k-means clustering algorithm.

Table 4.4. Coordinates of the dimensions studied.

	F1	F2	F3	F4	F5	F6	F7	F8	F9
Dim 1	1,495	-1,459	-0,762	-0,402	0,051	0,238	0,109	0,074	-0,013
Dim 2	1,068	0,599	-0,835	0,320	-0,494	-0,298	-0,042	0,004	-0,019
Dim 3	1,360	0,542	0,422	0,026	-0,317	0,446	-0,048	-0,089	-0,017
Dim 4	2,772	0,826	0,175	-0,186	-0,178	-0,001	-0,012	0,052	0,060
Dim 5	4,846	0,454	0,077	0,015	0,592	-0,125	-0,068	-0,016	-0,016
Dim 6	-1,402	2,262	0,445	-0,021	0,050	-0,136	0,167	-0,027	-0,010
Sun 7	-3,744	0,029	0,417	-0,767	-0,037	-0,107	-0,098	0,060	-0,016
Sun 8	-4,522	0,967	-0,626	0,504	0,330	0,199	-0,047	0,016	0,015
Sun 9	-1,525	-2,126	-0,164	-0,188	0,059	-0,166	0,019	-0,147	0,020
Sun 10	-0,347	-2,093	0,852	0,699	-0,054	-0,051	0,019	0,073	-0,005

Applying the k-means algorithm to the subspace defined by the PCA enabled us to identify groups of CSP dimensions where the dimensions in each group share the same properties. The most representative number of groups (k = 3) for this sample was deduced from the intra-class variances using the 'Elbow-Method' (**Figure 4.3**).

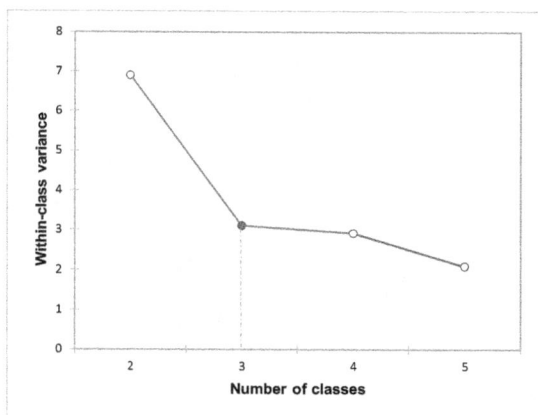

Figure 4.3. Intra-class variance as a function of the number of classes.

Based on the distances of each dimension from the defined centroids, the components (Dimensions) of the three groups were identified as follows (**Table 4.5**):

$G_1 = \{Dim_1 ; Dim_9 ; Dim_{10}\}$; $G_2 = \{Dim_2 ; Dim_3 ; Dim_4 ; Dim_5\}$; $G_3 = \{Dim_6$ $Dim_7 ; Dim_8\}$

Table 4.5. Classification of dimensions into 3 groups using the K-means algorithm.

Observation	Class	Distance to barycenter
Dim 1	1	1,678
Dim 2	2	1,444
Dim 3	2	1,153
Dim 4	2	0,342
Dim 5	2	2,339
Dim 6	3	2,168
Sun 7	3	1,179
Sun 8	3	1,305
Sun 9	1	1,419
Sun 10	1	0,298

Having defined the 3 groups of dimensions, it is now possible to represent them graphically on the PCA plan (**Figure 4.4**). This representation clearly shows the perimeters of each group and the dimensions included.

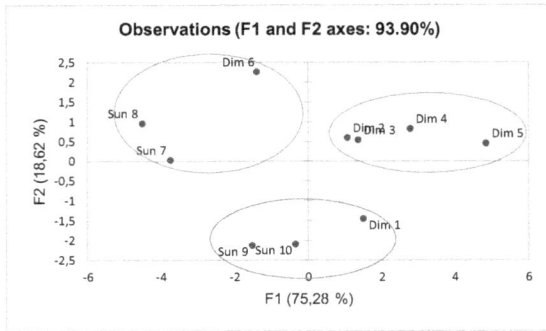

Figure 4.4. Visualisation of the groups resulting from the k-means algorithm.

The results obtained will be capitalised on to calculate PSC scores by group of dimensions in order to better lead to PSC improvement plans in hospital establishments.

c. Deduction of CS maturity levels P

The combined PCA/K-means approach shows that the dimensions of PSC can be grouped into three groups that can be described as macro-dimensions. These are labelled according to the characteristics shared by their constituent dimensions:

- MD_1 = Hospital level dimensions= {Dim1; Dim9; Dim10};

- MD_2 = Unit level dimensions= {Dim2; Dim3; Dim4; Dim5};

- MD_3 = Outcome dimensions = {Dim6 ; Dim7 ; Dim8}.

In addition, a closer look at the results shows that each macro-dimension can be linked to a PSC player who has a key role in promoting it. In this sense, Hospital level dimensions (MD₁) are linked to managers. Unit level dimensions (MD₂) are linked to employees. Outcome dimensions (MD₃) are linked to both managers and employees. This "macro-dimensions / SSC players" association helps to design a new model of SSC maturity, the immediate interest of which is that it makes it possible to highlight an action plan to improve the problematic macro-dimensions (scores $\leq 50\%$). In addition, the 3 macro-dimensions obtained contribute in turn to the deduction of the levels of maturity of the PSC for the 10 EHs (**Table 4.6**).

Table 4.6. Macro-dimensional scores and maturity levels of EHs.

	HE 1	HE 2	HE 3	HE 4	HE 5	HE 6	HE 7	HE 8	HE 9	HE 10
MD_1	40,1	70,5	56,7	42,6	43,2	69,9	40	43,8	31,8	55,9
MD_2	66,8	67,3	54,3	69,5	59,9	66,8	61,8	55	36,1	67,3
MD_3	48,8	21,9	29,5	43,2	38,9	28,8	41,8	33,7	17,4	34,1
Level of maturity	UD	UD	UD	UD	UD	UD	UD	UD	ND	UD
(ND) Undeveloped PSC (UD) Underdeveloped PSC (D) Developed PSC										

4.2.3. Discussions

a. Macro-dimensional CS scores P

This study was carried out to assess PSC in EHs with the aim of proposing a new approach to the mixed assessment of PSC. To this end, PSC was assessed in 10 HCTs using the HSOPSC questionnaire. The response rate, which reached 69%, testifies to the considerable involvement of healthcare professionals in this study. This response rate is considered satisfactory by several authors (Özcan et al. 2020; Tlili et al. 2020).

The macro-dimensional scores presented in **Table 4.6** show that the level of maturity of the PSC is underdeveloped for all the DHs except for EH9, where it was found to be undeveloped. MD_3 was found to be problematic for all the EHs. For example, EH_2 , EH_3 , EH_6 and EH_9 have scores of 21.9%, 29.5%, 28.8% and 17.4%. This means that their management style is a major obstacle to efforts to improve PSC. Consequently, managers need to take steps to facilitate the development of PSC by demonstrating leadership and commitment to PS.

In addition, MD_1 and MD_2 are underdeveloped for all EHs. As a result, an overall strategy needs to be implemented that aims to create an environment in which staff can feel safe in reporting problems and errors. This environment is characterised by a learning culture based on transparency, reliability, open communication and a strengthened flow of information. Improving working conditions and recognising individual initiative are also seen as key factors in improving UMC.

b. CS maturity levels P

Note that in the grid in **Figure 4.2**, the levels of maturity of the SSC are deduced from the scores obtained on the macro-dimensions. Hence the mixed assessment (qualitative and quantitative) of the SSC. In addition, the advantage of presenting the levels in the form of a grid is that it makes it possible to indicate, from one level of the CSP, the possibilities offered for reaching the highest level (developed). In other words, the recommended PSC maturity grid is a real decision-making tool for promoting PSC within HEIs by acting in an optimised way on the macro-dimensions that are said to be problematic.

c. Other benefits of evaluating the SSC by simultaneous use of the decisional

and typological approaches

The method proposed in this chapter for the mixed evaluation of PSC (by merging the decisional and typological approaches) can also be capitalised on at the practical and academic levels:

- on a practical level, government authorities (i.e. the Ministry of Health) can use the results to establish a national reform policy to promote PHC in the NHS,

- From an academic point of view, the quantification of the levels of maturity of the CSP is, to our knowledge, a novelty for the deduction of a model with four levels of maturity. In fact, this quantification of CSP maturity levels makes it possible to overcome the difficulties associated with traditional practices of deducing maturity levels through interviews, observations, audits and documentary analyses.

In other words, capitalising on the association of macro-dimensions of the SSC and its players (managers and employees) makes it possible to design a model of SSC maturity typical of that proposed by (Daniellou, Simard and Boissière, 2011) which has the merit of having four levels (i.e. fatalistic, managerial, business and integrated). As a reminder, these four levels can be quantified directly from the macro-dimensional scores (**Figure 4.5**): $0.33 < WIw \leq 0.89$; $0.33 < WIM \leq 0.89$; $0.89 < SIw \leq 1$; $0.89 < SIM \leq 1$.

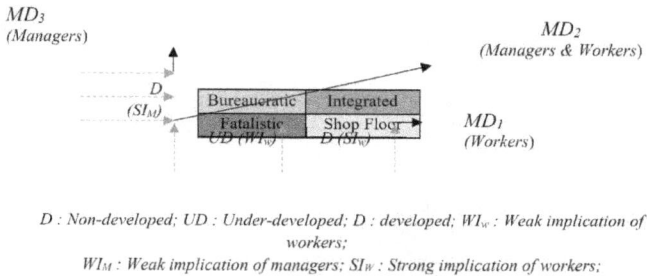

D : Non-developed; UD : Under-developed; D : developed; WI$_w$: Weak implication of workers;
WI$_M$: Weak implication of managers; SI$_w$: Strong implication of workers;

Figure 4.5. Adapted CSP maturity model.

4.3. Conclusion

The safety of healthcare has become a major concern in recent years. To improve care safety, healthcare organisations are putting in place initiatives influenced by PSC, which is assessed using questionnaires or maturity models.

However, these two approaches are often used separately, which has its limitations. This chapter presents a new mixed approach to PSC evaluation by combining principal component analysis (PCA) and the K-Means clustering algorithm.

This approach has been applied to healthcare establishments in Algeria, revealing challenges such as a predominant managerial vision and a blame culture. This highlights the importance of a participative culture, open communication and a non-punitive response to errors in improving patient safety.

Finally, we suggest a diachronic study to monitor the evolution of the care safety culture over time and develop models to predict its maturity.

Conclusion

Healthcare safety has become a major issue of public interest in recent years. This has led healthcare organisations to implement initiatives to improve safety behaviour. These are influenced by the culture of safety in healthcare, which can be assessed using questionnaires or maturity models.

It should be noted that these two evaluation approaches are often used separately, with certain limitations. All the literature specialising in PSC recommends the combined use of these approaches to overcome these limitations. In this context, Chapter 4 presented a new mixed PSC evaluation approach based on the combined use of PCA/K-Means methods. In this mixed approach, the dimensions of SSC were aggregated into macro-dimensions and then coupled with the SSC actors (managers and employees) that a new model of SSC maturity was highlighted.

Moreover, the application of this mixed approach to the evaluation of PSC to a group of Algerian HMEs has shown that their level of maturity is underdeveloped because of a managerial vision which takes precedence over the integrated vision. In addition, a blame culture is proving to be the main obstacle to the reporting of adverse events. This situation is exacerbated by the absence of an error reporting system and a lack of commitment to developing a learning culture. Therefore, a participatory culture based on open communication, non-punitive response to errors and transparency is more than necessary to improve patient safety in the EHs studied.

At the end of this study, we confirm that the answers provided to the two key questions raised in the introduction to this chapter have made it possible to resolve, on the one hand, the recurring problem of aggregating the dimensions of the SSC during its dimensional evaluation and, on the other hand, to quantify the levels of maturity of the SSC. There are many perspectives for this study. However, the one that seems urgent to us from an academic point of view is to carry out a *diachronic study* of mixed evaluation of PSC in a HE in order to get an idea of the development of this PSC within this HE. This diachronic study will undoubtedly give an idea of the progress made by a HE to promote its PSC. This information is extremely important for the development of *predictive models of the* maturity of the PSC that we are planning for future work.

a. *Prospects for the future*

There are still many innovative ideas in the field of PSC that need to be explored. Particularly at the fundamental level of PSC, where we plan to explore predictive models for integration into the typological approach to PSC in order to promote PSC maturity models, which to date suffer from the "static nature" of the maturity level. We would also point out that no explanation is provided by the CSS maturity models as to the progress that needs to be made in order to move towards the better levels of the CSP.

In this respect, we believe that the use of predictive models makes it possible to make CSP maturity models much more dynamic and, as a result, to provide information not only on the instantaneous maturity of the CSS but also on its trend over time. This is our primary ambition if we are to continue to contribute to the development of CSP.

Another perspective also concerns the four most popular CSP questionnaires (cf. chapter 3) where we plan to use *similarity methods* to be able to make comparisons between the different dimensions of these questionnaires. This very promising line of research requires the development of an entire ontology dedicated to the PSC, and within the framework of this ontology, any similarities between the PSC dimensions of the different questionnaires will undoubtedly make it possible to better generalise the dimensional evaluation of the PSC.

REFERENCES

ACSNI. 1993. *Third Report-Organising for Safety*. London, United Kingdom.

Antonsen, Stian. 2017. *Safety Culture: Theory, Method and Improvement*. Surrey, England: Ashgate Publishing Limited.

Ashcroft, D. M., C. Morecroft, D. Parker, and P. R. Noyce. 2005. "Safety Culture Assessment in Community Pharmacy: Development, Face Validity, and Feasibility of the Manchester Patient Safety Assessment Framework." *Quality and Safety in Health Care* 14(6):417-21.

Bandura, Albert. 1986. *Social Foundations of Thought and Action: Social Cognitive Theory*.

Behari, Niresh. 2019. "Assessing Process Safety Culture Maturity for Specialty Gas Operations: A Case Study." *Process Safety and Environmental Protection* 123:1-10. doi: 10.1016/j.psep.2018.12.012.

Benzer, Justin K., Mark Meterko, and Sara J. Singer. 2017. "The Patient Safety Climate in Healthcare Organizations (PSCHO) Survey: Short-Form Development." *Journal of Evaluation in Clinical Practice* 23(4):853-59.

Besnard, Denis, Ivan Boissières, François Daniellou, and Jesús Villena. 2018. *Safety Culture - From Understanding To Action*. Toulouse, France.

Boughaba, Assia, Salah Aberkane, Youcef-Oussama Fourar, and Mébarek Djebabra. 2019. "Study of Safety Culture in Healthcare Institutions: Case of an Algerian Hospital." *International Journal of Health Care Quality Assurance* 32(7):1081-97. doi: 10.1108/IJHCQA-09-2018-0229.

Braithwaite, Jeffrey, Jessica Herkes, Kristiana Ludlow, Luke Testa, and Gina Lamprell. 2017. "Association between Organisational and Workplace Cultures, and Patient Outcomes: Systematic Review." *BMJ Open* 7(11):e017708. doi: 10.1136/bmjopen-2017-017708.

Chen, I. Chi, Ng Lee Peng, Ng Hui Fuang, and Kuar Lok Sin. 2019. "Impacts of Job-Related Stress and Patient Safety Culture on Patient Safety Outcomes among Nurses in Taiwan." *International Journal of Healthcare Management* 0(0):1-9. doi: 10.1080/20479700.2019.1603419.

Christian, Michael S., Jill C. Bradley, J. Craig Wallace, and Michael J. Burke. 2009. "Workplace Safety: A Meta-Analysis of the Roles of Person and Situation Factors." *Journal of Applied Psychology* 94(5):1103-27. doi: 10.1037/a0016172.

Cleff, Thomas. 2014. "Univariate Data Analysis." Pp. 23-60 in *Exploratory Data Analysis in Business and Economics*. Cham: Springer International Publishing.

Cooper, D. M. 2002. "Safety Culture: A Model for Understanding and Quantifying a Difficult Concept." *Professional Safety* 47(6):30-36.

Cooper, Domnic. 2016. *Navigating the Safety Culture Construct: A Review of the Evidence*.

Cooper, M. D. 2000. "Towards a Model of Safety Culture." *Safety Science* 36(2):111-36. doi: 10.1016/S0925-7535(00)00035-7.

Cox, Sue, and Rhona Flin. 1998. "Safety Culture: Philosopher's Stone or Man of Straw?" *Work & Stress* 12(3):189-201. doi: 10.1080/02678379808256861.

Le Coze, Jean Christophe. 2019. "How Safety Culture Can Make Us Think." *Safety Science* 118(December 2018):221-29. doi: 10.1016/j.ssci.2019.05.026.

Daniellou, François, Marcel Simard, and Ivan Boissière. 2011. *Human and Organizational Factors of Safety: State of the Art*. Toulouse, France.

Daniellou, François, Marcel Simard, and Ivan Boissières. 2010. *Human and Organisational Factors in Industrial Safety*. Toulouse, France.

Ding, Chris, and Xiaofeng He. 2004. "Cluster Structure of K-Means Clustering via Principal Component Analysis." Pp. 414-18 in *Proceedings of the 21st International Confer-ence on Machine Learning*. Banff, Canada.

Dunstan, Elspeth, Jane Louise Cook, and Fiona Coyer. 2019. "Safety Culture in Intensive Care Internationally and in Australia: A Narrative Review of the Literature." *Australian Critical Care* 32(6):524-39. doi: 10.1016/j.aucc.2018.11.003.

DuPont[TM] . 2009. *Overview of DuPont ' s Safety Model and Sustainability Initiatives*. USA.

Famolaro, T., N. Yount, R. Hare, S. Thornton, K. Meadows, L. Fan, R. Birch, and J. Sorra. 2018. *Hospital Survey on Patient Safety Culture: 2018 User Database Report*. Rockville, MD. doi: AHRQ Publication No. 11-0030.

Fleming, Mark. 2000. *Safety Culture Maturity*. Edinburgh, UK.

Fleming, Mark. 2007. *Developing Safety Culture Measurement Tools and Techniques Based On Site Audits Rather Than Questionnaires.* Halifax.

Flin, R., K. Mearns, P. O'Connor, and R. Bryden. 2000. "Measuring Safety Climate: Identifying the Common Features." *Safety Science* 34(1-3):177-92. doi: 10.1016/S0925-7535(00)00012-6.

Foster, Patrick, and Stuart Hoult. 2013. "The Safety Journey: Using a Safety Maturity Model for Safety Planning and Assurance in the UK Coal Mining Industry." *Minerals* 3(1):59-72. doi: 10.3390/min3010059.

Fourar, Youcef Oussama, Wissal Benhassine, Assia Boughaba, and Mebarek Djebabra. 2020. "Contribution to the Assessment of Patient Safety Culture in Algerian Healthcare Settings: The ASCO Project." *International Journal of Healthcare Management* 0(0):1-10. doi: 10.1080/20479700.2020.1836736.

Fränti, Pasi, and Sami Sieranoja. 2019. "How Much Can K-Means Be Improved by Using Better Initialization and Repeats?" *Pattern Recognition* 93:95-112. doi: 10.1016/j.patcog.2019.04.014.

Fugas, Carla S., Sílvia A. Silva, and José L. Meliá. 2012. "Another Look at Safety Climate and Safety Behavior: Deepening the Cognitive and Social Mediator Mechanisms." *Accident Analysis & Prevention* 45:468-77. doi: 10.1016/j.aap.2011.08.013.

Gilbert, Claude, Benoît Journé, Hervé Laroche, and Corinne Bieder. 2018. *Safety Cultures, Safety Models.* edited by C. Gilbert, B. Journé, H. Laroche, and C. Bieder. Cham: Springer International Publishing.

Ginsburg, Liane, Debra Gilin, Deborah Tregunno, Peter G. Norton, Ward Flemons, and Mark Fleming. 2009. "Advancing Measurement of Patient Safety Culture." *Health Services Research* 44(1):205-24. doi: 10.1111/j.1475-6773.2008.00908.x.

Giorgi, Simona, Christi Lockwood, and Mary Ann Glynn. 2015. "The Many Faces of Culture: Making Sense of 30 Years of Research on Culture in Organization Studies." *Academy of Management Annals* 9(1):1-54. doi: 10.1080/19416520.2015.1007645.

Goh, Swee C., Christopher Chan, and Craig Kuziemsky. 2013. "Teamwork, Organizational Learning, Patient Safety and Job Outcomes." *International Journal of Health Care Quality Assurance* 26(5):420-32. doi: 10.1108/IJHCQA-05-2011-0032.

Goncalves Filho, Anastacio Pinto, and Patrick Waterson. 2018. "Maturity Models and Safety Culture: A Critical Review." *Safety Science* 105(February):192-211. doi: 10.1016/j.ssci.2018.02.017.

Goodrick, Delwyn. 2014. *Comparative Case Studies.* Italy.

Granel, Nina, Josep Maria Manresa-Domínguez, Carolina Eva Watson, Rebeca Gómez-Ibáñez, and Maria Dolors Bernabeu-Tamayo. 2020. "Nurses' Perceptions of Patient Safety Culture: A Mixed-Methods Study." *BMC Health Services Research* 20(1):1-9. doi: 10.1186/s12913-020-05441-w.

Griffin, Mark A., and Matteo Curcuruto. 2016. "Safety Climate in Organizations." *Annual Review of Organizational Psychology and Organizational Behavior* 3(1):191-212. doi: 10.1146/annurev-orgpsych-041015-062414.

Griffin, Mark A., and Andrew Neal. 2000. "Perceptions of Safety at Work: A Framework for Linking Safety Climate to Safety Performance, Knowledge, and Motivation." *Journal of Occupational Health Psychology* 5(3):347-58. doi: 10.1037/1076-8998.5.3.347.

Guldenmund, F. W. 2000. "The Nature of Safety Culture: A Review of Theory and Research." *Safety Science* 34(1-3):215-57. doi: 10.1016/S0925-7535(00)00014-X.

Guldenmund, Frank W. 2010. "Understanding and Exploring Safety Culture." Uitgeverij Boxpress, Oisterwijk, Delft, Netherlands.

Hadef, Hefaidh, and Mébarek Djebabra. 2019a. "PCA-I and AHP Methods: Unavoidable Arguments in Accident Scenario Classification." *Journal of Failure Analysis and Prevention* 19(2):496-503. doi: 10.1007/s11668-019-00625-x.

Hadef, Hefaidh, and Mébarek Djebabra. 2019b. "Proposal Method for the Classification of Industrial Accident Scenarios Based on the Improved Principal Components Analysis (Improved PCA)." *Production Engineering* 13(1):53-60. doi: 10.1007/s11740-018-0859-3.

Halligan, Michelle, and Aleksandra Zecevic. 2011. "Safety Culture in Healthcare: A Review of Concepts, Dimensions, Measures and Progress." *BMJ Quality & Safety* 20(4):338-43. doi: 10.1136/bmjqs.2010.040964.

Hefaidh, Hadef, and Djebabra Mébarek. 2020. "Using Fuzzy-Improved Principal Component Analysis (PCA-IF) for Ranking of Major Accident Scenarios." *Arabian Journal for Science and Engineering* 45(3):2235-45. doi: 10.1007/s13369-019-04233-7.

Heroual, N., F. Azza, S. Bouras, K. Madi, and L. Houti. 2016. "Approche de Mise En Place d'une Démarche d'évaluation de La Qualité Des Soins Dans Un Hôpital Spécialisé En Oncologie Dans l'Ouest Algérien, Oran, Algérie." *Journal of Epidemiology and Public Health* 64:S241-42. doi: 10.1016/j.respe.2016.06.269.

Hodgen, A., L. Ellis, K. Churruca, and M. Bierbaum. 2017. *Safety Culture Assessment in Health Care: A Review of the Literature on Safety Culture Assessment Modes*. Sydney, Australia.

Hudson, Patrick. 2007. "Implementing a Safety Culture in a Major Multi-National." *Safety Science* 45(6):697-722. doi: 10.1016/j.ssci.2007.04.005.

INSAG. 1986. *Summary Report on the Post-Accident Review Meeting on the Chernobyl Accident (Safety Series 75-INSAG-1)*. Vienna: International Atomic Energy Agency.

Karamizadeh, Sasan, Shahidan M. Abdullah, Azizah A. Manaf, Mazdak Zamani, and Alireza Hooman. 2013. "An Overview of Principal Component Analysis." *Journal of Signal and Information Processing* 04(03):173-75. doi: 10.4236/jsip.2013.43B031.

Kines, Pete, Jorma Lappalainen, Kim Lyngby Mikkelsen, Espen Olsen, Anders Pousette, Jorunn Tharaldsen, Kristinn Tómasson, and Marianne Törner. 2011. "Nordic Safety Climate Questionnaire (NOSACQ-50): A New Tool for Diagnosing Occupational Safety Climate." *International Journal of Industrial Ergonomics* 41(6):634-46. doi: 10.1016/j.ergon.2011.08.004.

Kirwan, Barry, Tom Reader, and Anam Parand. 2019. "The Safety Culture Stack - the next Evolution of Safety Culture?" *Safety and Reliability* 0(0):1-18. doi: 10.1080/09617353.2018.1556505.

Kohn, Linda T., Janet M. Corrigan, and S. Molla. 1999. *To Err Is Human*. Washington, D.C. doi: 10.1017/S095026880100509X.

Kottner, Jan, and David L. Streiner. 2010. "Internal Consistency and Cronbach's α: A Comment on Beeckman et al. (2010)." *International Journal of Nursing Studies* 47(7):926-28. doi: 10.1016/j.ijnurstu.2009.12.018.

Lardner, R., M. Fleming, and P. Joyner. 2002. "Towards a Mature Safety Culture." Pp. 635-42 in *Hazards Xvi: Analysing the Past, Planning the Future*. Manchester, UK.

Lee, Yii Ching, Shao Jen Weng, James O. Stanworth, Liang Po Hsieh, and Hsin Hung Wu. 2015. "Identifying Critical Dimensions and Causal Relationships of Patient Safety Culture in Taiwan." *Journal of Medical Imaging and Health Informatics* 5(5):995-1000. doi: 10.1166/jmihi.2015.1482.

Leggat, Sandra G., and Cathy Balding. 2018. "Effective Quality Systems: Implementation in Australian Public Hospitals." *International Journal of Health Care Quality Assurance* 31(8):1044-57. doi: 10.1108/IJHCQA-02-2017-0037.

Listyowardojo, Tita Alissa, Xiaoling Yan, Stephen Leyshon, Bobbie Ray-Sannerud, Xin Yan Yu, Kai Zheng, and Tao Duan. 2017. "A Safety Culture Assessment by Mixed Methods at a Public Maternity and Infant Hospital in China." *Journal of Multidisciplinary Healthcare* Volume 10:253-62. doi: 10.2147/JMDH.S136943.

Lund, J., and L. E. Aarø. 2004. *Accident Prevention. Presentation of a Model Placing Emphasis on Human, Structural and Cultural Factors*. Vol. 42.

María R. Calingo, Luís. 1996. "The Evolution of Strategic Quality Management." *International Journal of Quality & Reliability Management* 13(9):19-37. doi: 10.1108/02656719610150597.

McArdle, D., N. Burns, and A. Ireland. 2003. "Attitudes and Beliefs of Doctors towards Medication Error Reporting." *International Journal of Health Care Quality Assurance* 16(7):326-33. doi: 10.1108/09526860310499981.

Mouda, Mohammed, Mébarek Djebabra, Wafa Boulagouas, and Makhlouf Chati. 2016. "Proposal for an Evaluation Method for the Performance of Work Procedures." *Safety and Health at Work* 7(4):299-306. doi: 10.1016/j.shaw.2016.04.007.

Moumtzoglou, Anastasius. 2010. "Factors That Prevent Physicians Reporting Adverse Events." *International Journal of Health Care Quality Assurance* 23(1):51-58. doi: 10.1108/09526861011010677.

Noort, Mark C., Tom W. Reader, Steven Shorrock, and Barry Kirwan. 2016. "The Relationship between National Culture and Safety Culture: Implications for International Safety Culture Assessments." *Journal of Occupational and Organizational Psychology* 89(3):515-38. doi: 10.1111/joop.12139.

Occelli, P., J. L. Quenon, M. Kret, S. Domecq, F. Delaperche, O. Claverie, B. Castets-Fontaine, R. Amalberti, Y. Auroy, P. Parneix, and P. Michel. 2013. "Validation of the French Version of the Hospital Survey on Patient Safety Culture Questionnaire." *International Journal for Quality in Health Care* 25(4):459-68. doi: 10.1093/intqhc/mzt047.

Occelli, Pauline. 2018. "Measuring and Improving the Safety Climate of Care in French Health Establishments." University of Lyon 1.

Özcan, Taner Hasan, Sıdıka Kaya, and Mesut Teleş. 2020. "Evaluating Patient Safety Culture at a Private Hospital." *International Journal of Healthcare Management* 0(0):1-10. doi: 10.1080/20479700.2020.1755806.

Palese, Luigi Leonardo. 2018. "A Random Version of Principal Component Analysis in Data Clustering." *Computational Biology and Chemistry* 73:57-64. doi: 10.1016/j.compbiolchem.2018.01.009.

Parker, Dianne, Matthew Lawrie, and Patrick Hudson. 2006. "A Framework for Understanding the Development of Organisational Safety Culture." *Safety Science* 44(6):551-62. doi: 10.1016/j.ssci.2005.10.004.

Pattison, Jill, and Theresa Kline. 2015. "Facilitating a Just and Trusting Culture." *International Journal of Health Care Quality Assurance* 28(1):11-26. doi: 10.1108/IJHCQA-05-2013-0055.

Paulk, Mark C., Bill Curtis, Mary Beth Chrissis, and Charles V Weber. 1993. *Capability Maturity Model for Software, Version 1.1.* Carnegie-Mellon, Pennsylvania.

Penkova, T. G. 2017. "Principal Component Analysis and Cluster Analysis for Evaluating the Natural and Anthropogenic Territory Safety." Pp. 99-108 in *Procedia Computer Science.* Vol. 112. Elsevier B.V.

Pronovost, Peter J., Denise M. Cardo, Christine A. Goeschel, Sean M. Berenholtz, Sanjay Saint, and John A. Jernigan. 2011. "A Research Framework for Reducing Preventable Patient Harm." *Clinical Infectious Diseases* 52(4):507-13. doi: 10.1093/cid/ciq172.

Pullen, William. 2007. "Should We Have a Universal Model for HPT." *Performance Improvement* 46(4):9-16. doi: 10.1002/pfi.

Pumar-Méndez, María J., Moira Attree, and Ann Wakefield. 2014. "Methodological Aspects in the Assessment of Safety Culture in the Hospital Setting: A Review of the Literature." *Nurse Education Today* 34(2):162-70. doi: 10.1016/j.nedt.2013.08.008.

Rabbani, Fauziah, S. M. Wasim Jafri, Farhat Abbas, Firdous Jahan, Nadir Ali Syed, Gregory Pappas, Syed Iqbal Azam, Mats Brommels, and Göran Tomson. 2009. "Culture and Quality Care Perceptions in a Pakistani Hospital." *International Journal of Health Care Quality Assurance* 22(5):498-513. doi: 10.1108/09526860910975607.

Reason, James. 1998. "Achieving a Safe Culture: Theory and Practice." *Work & Stress* 12(3):293-306. doi: 10.1080/02678379808256868.

Reiman, Teemu, and Carl Rollenhagen. 2014. "Does the Concept of Safety Culture Help or Hinder Systems Thinking in Safety?" *Accident Analysis & Prevention* 68:5-15. doi: 10.1016/j.aap.2013.10.033.

Reis, Cláudia Tartaglia, Sofia Guerra Paiva, and Paulo Sousa. 2018. "The Patient Safety Culture: A Systematic Review by Characteristics of Hospital Survey on Patient Safety Culture Dimensions." *International Journal for Quality in Health Care* 30(9):660-77. doi: 10.1093/intqhc/mzy080.

Roney, Linda, Catherine Sumpio, Audrey M. Beauvais, and Eileen R. O'Shea. 2017. "Describing Clinical Faculty Experiences with Patient Safety and Quality Care in Acute Care Settings: A Mixed Methods Study." *Nurse Education Today* 49:45-50. doi: 10.1016/j.nedt.2016.11.014.

Sabry, Hend Aly, Mona Adel Soliman, Hafez Mahmoud Bazaraa, and Amira Aly Hegazy. 2020. "Improving Patient Safety at Pediatric Intensive Care Units: Exploring Healthcare Providers' Perspective." *International Journal of Healthcare Management* 0(0):1-6. doi: 10.1080/20479700.2020.1726032.

Schein, Edgar. H. 1992. *Organizational Culture and Leadership.* San Francisco: Jossey-Bass.

Schein, Edgar. H., and Peter Schein. 2017. *Organizational Culture and Leadership*. 5th Editio. New Jersey, USA: John Wiley & Sons.

Shaw-Taylor, Yoku. 2014. "Making Quality Improvement Programs More Effective." *International Journal of Health Care Quality Assurance* 27(4):264-70. doi: 10.1108/IJHCQA-02-2013-0017.

Shirali, Gh. A., M. Shekari, and K. A. Angali. 2016. "Quantitative Assessment of Resilience Safety Culture Using Principal Components Analysis and Numerical Taxonomy: A Case Study in a Petrochemical Plant." *Journal of Loss Prevention in the Process Industries* 40:277-84. doi: 10.1016/j.jlp.2016.01.007.

Silbey, Susan S. 2009. "Taming Prometheus: Talk About Safety and Culture." *Annual Review of Sociology* 35(1):341-69. doi: 10.1146/annurev.soc.34.040507.134707.

Silva, Sílvia, Maria Luísa Lima, and Conceição Baptista. 2004. "OSCI: An Organisational and Safety Climate Inventory." *Safety Science* 42(3):205-20. doi: 10.1016/S0925-7535(03)00043-2.

Speroff, T., S. Nwosu, R. Greevy, M. B. Weinger, T. R. Talbot, R. J. Wall, J. K. Deshpande, D. J. France, E. W. Ely, H. Burgess, J. Englebright, M. V. Williams, and R. S. Dittus. 2010. "Organisational Culture: Variation across Hospitals and Connection to Patient Safety Climate." *Quality and Safety in Health Care* 19(6):592-96. doi: 10.1136/qshc.2009.039511.

Stemn, Eric, Carmel Bofinger, David Cliff, and Maureen E. Hassall. 2019. "Examining the Relationship between Safety Culture Maturity and Safety Performance of the Mining Industry." *Safety Science* 113(December 2018):345-55. doi: 10.1016/j.ssci.2018.12.008.

Tlili, Mohamed Ayoub, Wiem Aouicha, Mohamed Ben Rejeb, Jihene Sahli, Mohamed Ben Dhiab, Souad Chelbi, Ali Mtiraoui, Houyem Said Laatiri, Thouraya Ajmi, Chekib Zedini, and Manel Mallouli. 2020. "Assessing Patient Safety Culture in 18 Tunisian Adult Intensive Care Units and Determination of Its Associated Factors: A Multi-Center Study." *Journal of Critical Care* 56:208-14. doi: 10.1016/j.jcrc.2020.01.001.

Vierendeels, Geert, Genserik Reniers, Karolien van Nunen, and Koen Ponnet. 2018. "An Integrative Conceptual Framework for Safety Culture: The Egg Aggregated Model (TEAM) of Safety Culture." *Safety Science* 103(September 2017):323-39. doi: 10.1016/j.ssci.2017.12.021.

Vogus, Timothy J., and Kathleen M. Sutcliffe. 2007. "The Safety Organizing Scale: Development and Validation of a Behavioral Measure of Safety Culture in Hospital Nursing Units." *Medical Care* 45(1):46-54. doi: 10.1097/01.mlr.0000244635.61178.7a.

Vu, Trang, and Helen De Cieri. 2014. *Safety Culture and Safety Climate Definitions Suitable for a Regulator: A Systematic Literature Review*. Caulfield East, Australia.

Wendler, Roy. 2012. "The Maturity of Maturity Model Research: A Systematic Mapping Study." *Information and Software Technology* 54(12):1317-39. doi: 10.1016/j.infsof.2012.07.007.

Westrum, Ron. 1993. "Cultures with Requisite Imagination." Pp. 401-16 in *Verification and Validation of Complex Systems: Human Factors Issues*. Berlin, Heidelberg: Springer Berlin Heidelberg.

Westrum, Ron. 2004. "A Typology of Organisational Cultures." *Quality and Safety in Health Care* 13:22-27. doi: 10.1136/qshc.2003.009522.

Wischet, Werner, and Claudia Schusterschitz. 2009. "Quality Management and Safety Culture in Medicine - Do Standard Quality Reports Provide Insights into the Human Factor of Patient Safety?" *German Medical Science* 7:1-8. doi: 10.3205/000089.

Xuanyue, Mao, Nie Yanli, Cui Hao, Jia Pengli, and Zhang Mingming. 2013. "Literature Review Regarding Patient Safety Culture." *Journal of Evidence-Based Medicine* 6(1):43-49. doi: 10.1111/jebm.12020.

Yousefi, Yadolah, Mehdi Jahangiri, Alireza Choobineh, Hamidreza Tabatabaei, Sareh Keshavarzi, Ali Shams, and Younes Mohammadi. 2016. "Validity Assessment of the Persian Version of the Nordic Safety Climate Questionnaire (NOSACQ-50): A Case Study in a Steel Company." *Safety and Health at Work* 7(4):326-30. doi: 10.1016/j.shaw.2016.03.003.

Zhu, Changsheng, Christian Uwa Idemudia, and Wenfang Feng. 2019. "Improved Logistic Regression Model for Diabetes Prediction by Integrating PCA and K-Means Techniques." *Informatics in Medicine Unlocked* 17(April):100179. doi: 10.1016/j.imu.2019.100179.

Zohar, Dov. 2010. "Thirty Years of Safety Climate Research: Reflections and Future Directions." *Accident Analysis & Prevention* 42(5):1517-22. doi: 10.1016/j.aap.2009.12.019.

Zohar, Dov, and Tal Polachek. 2014. "Discourse-Based Intervention for Modifying Supervisory Communication as Leverage for Safety Climate and Performance Improvement: A Randomized Field Study." *Journal of Applied Psychology* 99(1):113-24. doi: 10.1037/a0034096.

Appendix 1 (Questionnaire used to assess the CSS)

Section 1
Q1- Are you?
a. Man b. Woman
Q2- How old are you?
a. 20 - 30 years b. 31 - 40 years c. 41 - 50 years d. Older than 51years
Q3- How long have you worked in this hospital?
a. Less than 1 year b. 2 - 10 years c. 11 - 20 years d. 21 years or more
Q4- What is your professional category in this hospital?
....
Q5- What is your contract of employment?
a. Intern b. Fixed Duration Contract (FDC) c. Undetermined Duration Contract (UDC) d. Permanent

Section 2	SD	D	N	A	SA
Dim 1 - Overall perceptions of patient safety					
Q1 (-) : It is just by chance that more serious mistakes do not happen around here					
Q2 : Patient safety is never sacrificed to get more work done					
Q3 (-) : We have patient safety problems in this unit					
Q4 : Our procedures and systems are good at preventing errors from happening					
Dim 2 - Frequency of events reported					
Q5 : When a mistake is made, but is caught and corrected before affecting the patient, it is reported					
Q6 : When a mistake is made, but has no potential to harm the patient, it is reported					
Q7 : When a mistake is made that could harm the patient, but does not, it is reported					
Dim 3 - Supervisor/manager expectations and actions promoting safety					
Q8 : My supervisor says a good word when he/she sees a job done according to established patient safety procedures					
Q9: My supervisor seriously considers staff suggestions for improving patient safety					
Q10 (-) : Whenever pressure builds up, my supervisor wants us to work faster, even if it means taking shortcuts					
Q11 (-) : My supervisor overlooks patient safety problems that happen over and over					
Dim 4 - Organizational learning-continuous improvement					
Q12 : We are actively doing things to improve patient safety					
Q13: Mistakes have led to positive changes here					
Q14 : After we make changes to improve patient safety, we evaluate their effectiveness					
Q15 : We are given feedback about changes put into place based on event reports					
Q16: In this unit, we discuss ways to prevent errors from happening again					
Dim 5 - Teamwork within hospital units					
Q17 : People support one another in this unit					
Q18 : When a lot of work needs to be done quickly, we work together as a team to get the work done					
Q19: In this unit, people treat each other with respect					
Q20 : When one area in this unit gets really busy, others help out					
Dim 6 - Communication openness					
Q21: Staff will freely speak up if they see something that may negatively affect patient care					
Q22: Staff feel free to question the decisions or actions of those with more authority					
Q23(-): Staff are afraid to ask questions when something does not seem right					
Dim 7 - Non-punitive response to error					
Q24 (-): Staff feel like their mistakes are held against them					
Q25 (-): When an event is reported, it feels like the person is being written up, not the problem					
Q26 (-): Staff worry that mistakes they make are kept in their personnel file					
Dim 8 - Staffing					
Q27 : We have enough staff to handle the workload					
Q28 (-): Staff in this unit work longer hours than is best for patient care					
Q29 (-) : We work in 'crisis mode' trying to do too much, too quickly					
Dim 9 - Management support for patient safety					
Q30: Hospital management provides a work climate that promotes patient safety					
Q31: The actions of hospital management show that patient safety is a top priority					
Q32(-) :Hospital management seems interested in patient safety only after an adverse event happens					
Dim 10 - Teamwork across hospital units					
Q33 (-): Hospital units do not coordinate well with each other					
Q34 (-) : Things 'fall between the cracks' when transferring patients from one unit to another					
Q35: There is good cooperation among hospital units that need to work together					
Q36 (-): Important patient care information is often lost during shift changes					
Q37 (-): It is often unpleasant to work with staff from other hospital units					
Q38 (-): Problems often occur in the exchange of information across hospital units					

(-) : For negatively worded items, the percentage of positive response is the combined percentage of respondents within a hospital who answered 'Strongly disagree' or 'Disagree', because a negative answer on a negatively worded item indicates a positive response.
Strongly disagree (SD), disagree (D), neutral (N), agree (A) and strongly agree (SA).

Appendix 2 (Graphical representation of CSS dimensional scores)

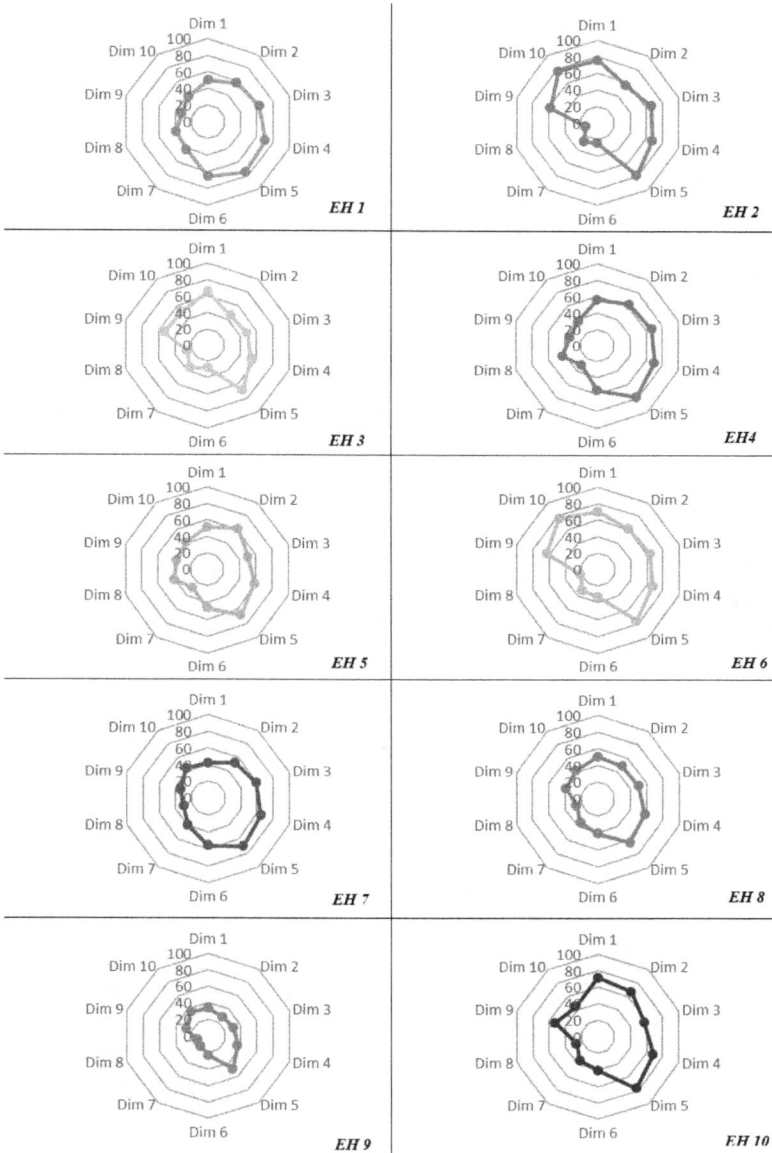

EH 1

EH 2

EH 3

EH 4

EH 5

EH 6

EH 7

EH 8

EH 9

EH 10

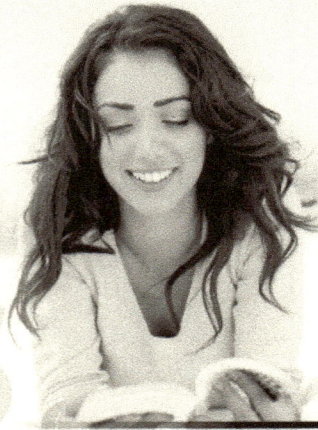

www.ingramcontent.com/pod-product-compliance
Lightning Source LLC
Chambersburg PA
CBHW021120210326

41598CB00017B/1511